Overcoming Common Problems

Coeliac Disease
What you need to know
Second edition

ALEX GAZZOLA

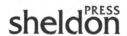

First published in Great Britain by Sheldon Press in 2011
An imprint of John Murray Press
A division of Hodder & Stoughton Ltd,
An Hachette UK company

This paperback edition published in 2020

1

This book is for information or educational purposes only and is not intended
to act as a substitute for medical advice or treatment. Any person with a
condition requiring medical attention should consult a qualified medical
practitioner or suitable therapist.

A CIP catalogue record for this title is available from the British Library

Paperback ISBN 9781529381085
eBook ISBN 9781529346848

Typeset by Cenveo® Publisher Services.

Printed and bound in Great Britain by Clays Ltd, Elcograf S.p.A.

John Murray Press policy is to use papers that are natural, renewable and
recyclable products and made from wood grown in sustainable forests. The
logging and manufacturing processes are expected to conform to the environmental regulations of the country of origin.

John Murray Press
Carmelite House
50 Victoria Embankment
London EC4Y 0DZ

www.sheldonpress.co.uk

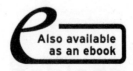

Contents

Foreword

Long before I was diagnosed with coeliac disease and even before I became the resident doctor on ITV's *This Morning*, I was particularly concerned with health issues that had a big impact on people's lives but weren't well known. I feel that it is my duty as a general practitioner to get to the root of people's problems and begin the process of healing, even though at times diagnosis and treatment can be complicated processes. This is why the widespread misunderstanding and confusion surrounding coeliac disease sparked such an interest in me.

I was appointed Health Ambassador for Coeliac UK in July 2007, just months before I received the MBE from Her Majesty the Queen, and relished the opportunity to work alongside a national charity doing such great work to support people with the condition and in raising awareness. Once I had learned more about its work I was keen to get involved and I haven't looked back since.

My position as Coeliac UK's Health Ambassador began to make clear to me the level of suffering that some people endure until they get an accurate diagnosis. I had never considered that the condition would have such a direct effect on my own life.

When I became ill it seemed impossible to me that the symptoms I was experiencing could be coeliac disease. As a doctor it is difficult to interpret your own symptoms objectively, so I became another coeliac who was misdiagnosed with irritable bowel syndrome (IBS). I was losing weight rapidly and was regularly gripped with terrible stomach pains and troublesome diarrhoea. Despite treatment for IBS my symptoms persisted, so I returned to my gastroenterologist, who performed a blood test and intestinal biopsy for coeliac disease. The disturbing factor for me was the not knowing – and although the positive diagnosis came as a shock, I was grateful to have answers.

My diagnosis reinforces my drive to raise awareness of coeliac disease and illustrates the importance of quick and accurate recognition of the condition. My work with Coeliac UK has been incredibly rewarding, and I have seen real growth in awareness of the condition, something to which I think *Coeliac Disease: What you need to know* will contribute.

Now that I am on a strict gluten-free diet for life, I realize how difficult it can sometimes be to stick to this, the only treatment for coeliac disease, and maintain the lifestyle I was used to. Even in the short time I've been diagnosed I've seen an improvement in restaurants and shops selling gluten-free food, but this does need to get better so that we can eat out without the worry.

One of the reasons I struggled to identify my own coeliac disease was the wide-ranging list of complaints that can be associated with it. Alex Gazzola's book addresses this by comprehensively listing the full spectrum of symptoms associated with coeliac disease in a step-by-step introduction to the condition as a whole.

To the casual reader, this book will be impressive because of the amount of interesting information available. To those who have coeliac disease it will provide a lifeline that allows them to allay their own fears while learning of the advances in medical research and the food industry in recent years. Diagnosis is the first challenge. There are half a million people living with symptoms in the UK who have not been diagnosed and are not even aware of how much better they could feel on a gluten-free diet.

It was a great honour to be asked to write the Foreword to such a thorough look into the world of this condition. Coeliac disease represents a confusing journey for so many people, and this book provides an accurate and supportive guide to help clear away the fog along the way.

Dr Chris Steele MBE
Health Ambassador, Coeliac UK

Acknowledgements

I am grateful to all those with coeliac disease or working with those with coeliac disease who have spoken to me about the condition since I started writing about it, and whose knowledge of and expertise in this fascinating illness has found its way in some form or other into this book. In particular, I'd like to thank Susan Cane, Dr William Dickey, Professor Alessio Fasano, Professor David Sanders – and Norma McGough, Kate Newman, Amy Peterson, Dr Chris Steele and all at Coeliac UK.

In addition, thanks to Michelle Berriedale-Johnson, Fiona Marshall and Eve Menezes Cunningham.

On a personal note, thanks and love to F, R and S.

Note to the reader

This book is designed to be as helpful and supportive as possible but cannot be used to diagnose or treat a medical condition, and neither is it intended as a substitute for professional advice. If you suspect you have a problem, consult a doctor.

Introduction

Coeliac disease hasn't always been with us because gluten hasn't always been with us.

For most of the 200,000 years during which we humans have been around to nourish ourselves, we've done so by foraging for vegetables, roots, fruits, nuts, leaves, grubs and insects – supplemented with the odd feast of scavenged or hunted meat.

Around 10,000 years ago, we observed that the watered seeds of plants could give life to new plants of the same kind, which in turn would grow, eventually to bear more seeds. From there, the leap to cultivating plant-based crops and building permanent bases around these new sources of food was a swift one. The hunter-gatherer lifestyle gave way to one of agriculture and settlement. The Neolithic agricultural revolution had begun.

Barley and ancient forms of wheat – einkorn, emmer – were cultivated first in the Fertile Crescent, and later more widely, as our ancestors migrated from the Middle East to China, Europe and beyond. The domestication of animals introduced their protein-rich products – milk, eggs – into our diets too. These were all novel foods to humans. Never underestimate the human capacity to adapt – it is why we are still flourishing – but not everyone's body could manage the transition so seamlessly. Food sensitivities began to emerge.

These intolerances are unlikely to have been considered new illnesses. Coeliac disease would have been looked upon much as any other severe, unpleasant disease characterized by the not unfamiliar symptoms of diarrhoea, wasting and general malaise common at the time, due to any number of bacterial infections and gastrointestinal upsets that would routinely have shortened lives. We must assume deaths related to coeliac disease – especially in the young – continued grimly for many years.

It was a Greek physician, Aretaeus of Cappadocia, who first distinguished – and named – coeliac disease in the first century A.D. 'If the stomach be irretentive of the food and if it pass through undigested and crude, and nothing ascends into the body, we call such persons coeliacs', he was found to have written, when his medical texts were translated into English in the nineteenth century. (The word 'coeliac' was derived from Aretaeus' use of the Greek word *koiliakós*, meaning 'suffering in the bowels'.) It is remarkable how astutely he recognized the poor absorption of nutrition that characterizes classical coeliac disease.

Aretaeus had also observed that 'bread is rarely suitable for giving strength', but little progress was made on the dietary connection until Dr Matthew Baillie, an early nineteenth-century physician, noted that some of his coeliac patients 'have appeared to derive considerable advantage from living almost entirely upon rice'. Yet even this observation was largely overlooked, and it wasn't until the late nineteenth century that paediatrician Samuel Gee, renowned lecturer in medicine at St Bart's Hospital, London, moved us a step forward.

'A kind of chronic indigestion which is met with in persons of all ages' was how Gee described the illness he dubbed the coeliac 'affection'. He wrote of the 'wasting, weakness and pallor' of patients and noted rightly that 'if the patient can be cured at all, it must be by means of diet'. He was almost there when he stated that 'the allowance of farinaceous [floury] food must be small', yet his diets were imperfect: they recommended meats and mussels but also thin slices of toast, and they disallowed fruit, vegetables and safe sources of starchy carbohydrate. There would have been improvements on such a lower-gluten diet, but not relief by any means.

Progress was patchy in subsequent decades. It was observed that non-diarrhoeal forms of coeliac disease could exist, and that there was a greater co-incidence among family members.

In 1924 the banana diet became popular. Introduced by American paediatrician Sidney Haas, who attempted it experimentally on several children whose health subsequently improved, the diet eliminated potatoes, breads and all cereals, and remained the treatment of choice for several decades, doubtlessly sparing lives. Haas believed it was the removal of carbohydrate that drove recuperation in coeliac patients, and he maintained this conviction long after it had been demonstrated that what was actually responsible was the restriction of wheat protein – that is, gluten.

The breakthrough

It was the insight of Dutch paediatrician Willem-Karel Dicke that led to this landmark discovery. It is widely related that he made the observation during the Second World War that coeliac children improved markedly when wheat and rye flours were unavailable and relapsed as soon as supplies were restored to the Netherlands. But he had, in fact, begun to suspect a link to wheat by the mid-1930s, after manipulating the diets of some of his young patients upon hearing anecdotal reports from mothers of the benefit to their children of a bread-free diet.

After years of research, development of his diet, and more formal studies, Dicke became convinced of the value to coeliacs of excluding wheat, and by the early 1950s he had shown that it was its protein – not carbohydrate – that triggered coeliac disease, a fact soon confirmed by other European researchers but that took longer to be accepted in America.

British physician John Paulley realized in 1954 that gluten eroded the architecture of the small intestinal lining, and that this damage could be at least partially reversed by avoiding gluten. In 1956, gastroenterologist Dr Margot Shiner developed a medical device that could be passed through the mouth, oesophagus and stomach and into the small intestine to allow the removal of samples of its lining. These could then be examined for any characteristic erosion. And so what became the diagnostic technique in the 1960s was developed: biopsy to look for damage, followed by a gluten-free diet, followed by another biopsy to look for improvement, followed by a gluten 'challenge', followed by another biopsy to check for the return of damage. This elaborate process, as unpleasant as it was for the patient, was considered necessary, given there could be other possible causes of intestinal lining inflammation and erosion.

Also in the 1960s, the hereditary nature of coeliac disease was established, as was gluten's link to the coeliac-related skin condition dermatitis herpetiformis. The Coeliac Society – now Coeliac UK – was founded.

The 1970s and 1980s were characterized by debate and research on the reason for coeliacs' gut sensitivity to gluten. Was it a toxin in the protein? An absent enzyme? Gradually it became recognized that coeliac disease was associated with so-called autoimmune conditions – diseases in which the body's immune system attacks its own tissues – such as type 1 diabetes and thyroid disease. And in the late 1980s and early 1990s, the theory of an immunological basis for coeliac disease was finally accepted: it too was an autoimmune disease, triggered by gluten and associated with particular gene types.

Blood tests to examine levels of antibodies associated with the disease could now be developed, paving the way towards more convenient ways of making the diagnosis of coeliac disease and reducing the need for multiple biopsies to just one. Population studies suggested a prevalence much higher than previously believed – closer to one in 100 than one in several thousand – and with that came the appreciation of a huge underdiagnosed population worldwide.

The current picture

Thanks to campaigning from coeliac charities, increased media coverage and the voices of coeliacs themselves, there is undoubtedly a greater awareness of coeliac disease and the gluten-free lifestyle. Specialist gluten-free foods have become widely available, and we have seen remarkable growth in this 'free from' sector. Food labelling is more precise.

Gastroenterologists (specialist gut doctors) now appreciate that coeliac disease manifests itself in a spectrum of symptoms – so much so that it should no longer be looked upon as solely a disease of the gut. Genetic advances – many beyond the scope of this book – continue worldwide. Clinical trials of a number of therapies are under way too, including enzyme pills, vaccines and other treatments. Within five or ten years, the lives of coeliacs could be transformed. A cure is not out of the question.

How this book will help

We are living in a time of nutritional information overload: never before have we been so bloated with advice on what, how and even when to eat – and why. Increase antioxidants to fight cancer. Reduce tomatoes to ease arthritis. Boost oily fish to relieve eczema. The evidence base for these and other claims like them varies considerably, but the public would be forgiven for thinking that there are any number of diseases that can definitively be treated through dietary manipulation alone. The truth is that there are few. Coeliac disease is one of them.

In writing *Coeliac Disease: What you need to know* I've taken what we currently know about the disease and tried to distil it into a slim but fact-filled volume. Essentially, it tells you how to find out whether you, or your child, need to avoid gluten, how to avoid gluten if one of you does need to, and how best to ensure a healthy gluten-free life.

It covers essentials such as testing and diagnosis – but if you've been diagnosed already and have been given a good grounding in coeliac disease from your dietitian or gastroenterologist, you can jump forward to the chapters on food labelling, diet and nutrition – including important changes to allergen and gluten-free labelling laws and the low FODMAP diet. The psychological and emotional impact of coeliac disease is usually given little coverage – a chapter here addresses that. Some of the more recent and exciting developments in coeliac disease are looked at in the final chapter. A comprehensive 'Useful addresses' section collates the useful associations and sources of information referred to throughout, many of which can offer answers to questions beyond the book's scope. Finally, the books listed in 'Further reading' provide additional sources of information.

The book, then, is aimed at several groups of people:

- those who suspect they may have the condition and want to find out more;
- adults or parents of children who have recently been diagnosed with the disease, and need a supportive, practical guide and convenient reference book;

- long-established coeliac patients who are interested in learning about the more recent developments, and how these may affect them.

Others, I hope, may also find the book useful: those eliminating gluten for other health or lifestyle reasons, loved ones of those with coeliac disease, student or qualified dietitians and doctors, health writers . . .

Note: the abbreviations CD (coeliac disease), GF (gluten free) and GFD (gluten-free diet) are used throughout. (The term 'gluten free' when used in specific relation to food labelling is not abbreviated.)

1

What coeliac disease is

Coeliac disease (CD) is characterized by chronic inflammation and erosion to the lining of the small intestine – the section of the digestive system that connects the stomach to the large intestine or colon and helps to digest and absorb food and nutrients – in genetically predisposed individuals.

The damage is caused by consuming gluten – a mix of proteins found in wheat, barley and rye, and therefore in many foods, such as breads, cakes and pastas, that contain them.

CD is not a food allergy, and neither is it accurate to call it a food intolerance. It is an autoimmune disease. Autoimmune diseases are those in which the body's immune system attacks its own tissues. In CD, these tissues are those of the gut – although other organs may well also be affected.

The disease is permanent and presently incurable, but symptoms can be resolved and damage reversed in virtually all cases when gluten is removed from the diet.

(Coeliac is pronounced *see-lee-ack* and is spelled 'celiac' in North America.)

Symptoms

CD can affect many organs and systems in the body, producing any number of a wide range of non-specific symptoms that vary in severity between patients.

Some people have few or no obvious symptoms.

Symptoms in adults

Among the possible symptoms are:

- digestive – diarrhoea, fatty stools, bloating, wind, abdominal pain, constipation, heartburn, indigestion, nausea, sickness, loss of appetite, weight loss

- nutritional – deficiency of iron (anaemia), vitamin B12, folic acid and other minerals and vitamins (caused by poor absorption of nutrients as a result of the damaged gut lining)
- skin and hair – mouth ulcers, dermatitis herpetiformis (an itchy and blistering skin rash), hair loss
- musculoskeletal – muscle wasting, muscle spasms, joint or muscle pain, osteopenia or osteoporosis (thinning or brittle bones), defective dental enamel
- nervous system – numbness, tingling in the hands or feet (neuropathy), seizures or epilepsy, unsteadiness or shaking (ataxia)
- reproductive – delayed puberty, low fertility, recurrent miscarriage, early menopause
- cardiovascular – irregular heartbeat, palpitations, breathlessness
- emotional – depression, anxiety, mood swings
- physical – pallor, tiredness or lethargy, poor growth.

Presentation of symptoms in adults

It used to be the case that the 'typical' adult coeliac patient presented with severe digestive complaints and strong signs of malnutrition, but while doctors still see such patients, these days they are no longer the norm.

Instead, the kinds of people who doctors see have vague, non-specific or non-serious complaints, such as mild tummy upsets, feelings of tiredness, unresolved irritable bowel syndrome (IBS) or a general sense of ill health.

Diarrhoea remains a common symptom, but it affects only around half of new patients, and it may be sporadic.

Other commonly reported symptoms are tiredness or lethargy (often caused by anaemia), weight loss, bloating and abdominal discomfort or pain. In fact, fatigue and anaemia are increasingly typical of new presentations of the disease.

Symptoms can come on so gradually that patients may not recognize that their health is slowly deteriorating. Often, when they do realize it, they may have only a vague sense of when the decline began.

Symptoms in babies and children

Infants and children can present with some of the complaints common to adults with CD, but typical symptoms generally include:

- digestive – diarrhoea or otherwise abnormal or pale stools, swollen tummy, low appetite or refusal to feed, vomiting, constipation
- emotional – behavioural problems, tearfulness, irritability
- physical – tiredness, signs of malnourishment, weak or wasted muscles, stunted growth or inability to gain weight.

Presentation of symptoms in children

Typical childhood CD is characterized by the onset of obvious symptoms at between six months and two years (i.e. soon after the usual introduction of grains), including pale diarrhoea, vomiting, swollen abdomen, muscle wasting, failure to gain weight, and general physical and emotional ill health.

Older children are more likely to have less severe digestive troubles, which may come and go. There may be delayed growth or puberty. There may be defects in tooth enamel, nutritional deficiencies and behavioural problems too.

Teenagers are more likely than other age groups (adults included) to show no symptoms at all, but any of the typical symptoms may present.

Prevalence

Screening studies suggest that around 1 per cent of Western populations has CD, though it varies by country and ethnicity.

However, only around 30 per cent of those with the disease in the UK are diagnosed – meaning 70 per cent of those with CD remain undetected. This represents almost 500,000 people.

Onset and diagnosis

CD can present at any point in life, from six months onwards well into old age.

Until only a decade ago it was believed that the detection of the disease in later life implied a long-standing undiagnosed case of CD, but new research has shown that this is not necessarily true. The disease can be triggered at any age, even after many years of gluten tolerance.

Peak age for diagnoses is among the under-tens and in those aged in their 40s – but increasing numbers are being diagnosed in older age.

Delayed diagnosis remains a significant problem, with many patients waiting over a decade after initially reporting symptoms.

Increased awareness among the medical profession and the general public means this picture is improving, however.

Susceptibility and risk factors

Thanks to ever more cutting-edge research, we have come to learn more about who is susceptible to CD and which factors determine whether you may develop it. However, the full picture is not yet clear.

Genetics

There is a strong genetic component to CD. If you have an identical twin with CD, there is at least a 70 per cent chance you will have it or develop it too. If a first-degree relative (parent, sibling, child) has the disease, you are ten times as likely as the general population to have it (a 10 per cent chance). If a second-degree relative (grandparent, aunt, uncle, nephew, niece) has CD, you are twice as likely as the general population to have it (a 2 per cent chance).

During the last decade scientists have unlocked more genetic secrets of CD, and we now know that virtually all people who develop the disease have one of two genetic tissue types, called HLA-DQ2 and HLA-DQ8. However, this is also true of around a third of the non-coeliac population, so clearly these genes are required, but not sufficient, for the development of CD.

Gluten and diet

Gluten must be present in the diet for CD to be expressed. Generally, the more gluten eaten, the more severe any symptoms, and possibly the greater the number of types of symptoms experienced.

In some cases, the quantity and type of gluten consumed could be involved in triggering the disease. There have been suggestions that modern cultivars of wheat could be more problematic than ancient and traditional gluten grains. The intake of highly processed white flour-based products and the widespread consumption of loaves made by the Chorleywood Bread Process – which drastically reduced dough fermentation times when it was introduced in the 1960s, and which deploys a number of enzymes and other processing aids – has been implicated too. The ideas remain disputed and unproven.

'Leaky gut'

Patients with CD are more likely to have a so-called leaky gut – that is, an intestinal lining that is more permeable than normal, and that allows incompletely digested food fragments, which are usually excluded from being absorbed, to pass through and potentially trigger an immune response.

Trigger events

For most people, there appears to be no clear reason or cause for the onset of symptoms of CD, but in others it seems connected to an obvious trigger event. It is possible that these events are involved in either triggering the disease itself or in inciting more obvious signs in existing CD that has been previously symptom-free. They include:

- a bout of severe stress
- pregnancy or childbirth
- food poisoning or gastroenteritis – often associated with overseas travel and perhaps with the use of antibiotics
- gastrointestinal surgery – again perhaps with antibiotics.

Disturbance of the gut bacteria population, which helps to maintain gut health, appears to be a common denominator in the obvious triggers. This could make the gut leakier and increase the likelihood of an immune response.

Other, unknown and subtler trigger events may also be involved. A trigger event may be required in all cases – perhaps with the exception of infants who develop CD soon after gluten introduction.

Sex

More women than men are diagnosed with CD, and while it is probable that this goes for undiagnosed cases too (since other autoimmune conditions tend to affect more women than men), it is possible that women are more likely to be diagnosed because they make more visits to their doctors. It may also be related to pregnancy, when immune function is altered.

Underlying autoimmunity

Patients with other autoimmune conditions are more likely to have CD. Around 3 per cent of the population have an autoimmune disease, and around 30 per cent of CD patients have at least one other autoimmune disease.

Type 1 diabetes (insulin-dependent diabetes)

Around 5-6 per cent of those with type 1 diabetes have CD.

Autoimmune liver disease

At least 5 per cent of those with one of the several types of autoimmune liver disease will have CD.

Autoimmune thyroid disease

Up to 7 per cent of those with thyroid disease may have CD.

Other autoimmune disease

There appear to be associations with other autoimmune conditions such as Sjögren's syndrome, inflammatory bowel diseases

(Crohn's disease and ulcerative colitis), psoriasis, Addison's disease and rheumatoid arthritis.

Genetic syndromes

People with Turner's syndrome, Williams' syndrome or Down's syndrome have an increased risk of CD – as do their first-degree relatives.

The spectrum of gluten-related disorders

Although CD was previously thought of as a 'black or white' disease – you either had it or you didn't – this is no longer seen as an accurate picture. We now consider a 'spectrum' of coeliac manifestations – and indeed of gluten-related disorders.

Symptomatic coeliac disease

This is characterized by clinically obvious symptoms attributable to gluten intake.

Classical coeliac disease

This is CD presenting with diarrhoea, malnutrition and weight loss or failure to thrive.

Non-classical coeliac disease

This is CD presenting with symptoms other than those related to poor absorption (i.e. diarrhoea and malnutrition).

Asymptomatic coeliac disease

This is CD in the absence of symptoms at initial diagnosis, and in which no subsequent symptomatic improvements are noted following the introduction of a gluten-free diet (GFD).

Potential coeliac disease

This term is used to describe a condition where a patient has a normal gut lining but is judged as being at increased risk of developing CD owing to positive blood tests.

Dermatitis herpetiformis

Dermatitis herpetiformis (DH) is an intensely itchy skin condition, characterized by blistery, reddened patches, usually on the elbows, knees, buttocks or scalp. It typically affects adults.

It is caused by gluten, and may be regarded as the skin manifestation of CD – although some see it as a separate condition. Patients may have 'classical' symptoms of CD, but most will not. Of this latter group, many are found to have damage to the gut lining or abnormal blood test results for CD when investigated.

Gluten ataxia

This is a neurological (nerve- and brain-related) form of gluten sensitivity, again considered by some a separate disorder from CD rather than a form of it.

Ataxia is loss of healthy muscular co-ordination. The symptoms include problems with walking and limb co-ordination, balance problems, speech problems, twitching, and poor control over eye movements.

Gluten ataxia (GA) is caused by damage to the part of the brain called the cerebellum, which is responsible for controlling these key functions. It can be present even in the absence of the gut lining damage associated with classical CD.

Gluten neuropathy

This is also a neurological form of gluten sensitivity. Peripheral neuropathy is nerve damage in the parts of the nervous system outside the spinal cord and brain. This is typically experienced as tingling and numbness in the hands and feet, and called sensory neuropathy. If there is difficulty in using the arms, hands, feet and legs, it is termed motor neuropathy.

Non-coeliac gluten sensitivity

Non-coeliac gluten sensitivity (NCGS) is the name that has been given to a condition with similar symptoms to those of CD (with a possible greater tendency towards non-gastrointestinal symptoms, such as tiredness, joint pain and headache) in which other forms of known reactions to gluten (such as CD and wheat allergy (WA)) have been ruled out. Patients with NCGS improve following the introduction of a GFD, but relapse when reintroducing gluten-containing foods. There is no gut lining damage in NCGS – and neither is the gut 'leakier'.

It is not known how many may have NCGS (estimates range from one in 200 to one in 16), how much gluten is sufficient to trigger symptoms, whether the condition is permanent or transient, whether it is hereditary or genetic, or what the long-term prognosis is.

It is controversial, because it remains unproven that gluten is in fact responsible for NCGS, leading some experts to argue that its name is inappropriate. It seems unclear to what degree the immune system is involved in NCGS – if at all. Some have speculated that wheat starches, non-gluten wheat proteins or other components of wheat may be the triggers. Others, that NCGS is in fact a 'pre-coeliac' condition.

In some patients, symptoms may resolve merely because of positive changes to the diet and nutrition following gluten elimination – more whole foods, fruit and vegetables, for instance.

The psychologically powerful placebo effect could be involved, whereby patients feel better on a GFD because they *expect* to feel better on a GFD, and this belief exerts a positive physiological impact. There is also the possibility of a nocebo effect, whereby patients feel worse when consuming gluten-containing foods that they have mistakenly come to believe harm them – and it is this that manifests the physical symptoms.

It may be that what we are calling NCGS turns out to be several distinct conditions or reactions – some defined and some as yet unknown.

Other gluten-related conditions

Other gluten-related conditions may be discovered. Links between gluten and schizophrenia, for instance, and gluten and epilepsy, are being explored.

The language of gluten

Confused by gluten-related terminology? It's an issue that can baffle lay persons and medical experts alike, with both susceptible to misusing expressions. Here is a list of additional terms, old and new, you may come across.

The expressions 'typical coeliac disease' and 'atypical coeliac disease' were once used to describe CD with and without symptoms of malabsorption respectively, but now 'classical coeliac disease' and 'non-classical coeliac disease' are preferred.

- 'Silent coeliac disease' is a former term for the now preferred 'asymptomatic coeliac disease'.
- 'Latent coeliac disease' once described various scenarios, including what we now call 'potential coeliac disease'.
- 'Coeliac sprue' is an outdated term for CD, still occasionally used in North America.
- 'Gluten-sensitive enteropathy' is a term for CD, often used among medics. It also describes gluten sensitivity in animals.
- 'Gluten allergy' strictly should only be used to denote a rapid-onset allergic reaction to gluten. It is a type of wheat allergy (allergies to other wheat proteins also occur).
- The term 'gluten intolerance' is common in conversation and has been used inaccurately to describe CD or NCGS, or other supposed or proposed responses to wheat or gluten. Because of this inconsistency, the term is discouraged.
- 'Gluten sensitivity' has been misused as a synonym for CD or as an umbrella term, and to describe reactions to gluten in the absence of CD or WA. In the last case, 'non-coeliac gluten sensitivity' is more suitable.

Gluten-related disorders is the correct umbrella term, incorporating CD, NCGS, DH, GA and WA.

The biology of coeliac disease

CD mainly affects the top section of the small intestine, a key part of the digestive system. In order to understand what happens in CD, we first need to understand how digestion works.

Digestion

Most food is of no use to the body in the form in which we consume it. In order for it to be of value, it must be broken down into smaller constituents that the body can absorb and reassemble – for instance, to build new cells or to nourish and fuel existing ones. The process of breaking down food is called digestion.

Digestion occurs in the digestive tract (or alimentary canal): the muscular tube that starts at your mouth, takes in the oesophagus (gullet or foodpipe), stomach, small and large intestines, and ends – nine or ten metres later – at your bottom.

The agents that help to break down the food into simpler molecules are called digestive enzymes. Many of the enzymes and chemicals needed for digestion are produced in the salivary glands, the liver, the gall bladder and the pancreas – vital organs, which together with the digestive tract make up the digestive system. Other enzymes are secreted by the cells lining the wall of the small intestine.

At around six or seven coiled metres, the small intestine consists of three connected parts – the duodenum, the jejunum and the ileum – and it is here that most digestion and absorption of food takes place. The upper sections of the small intestine – the duodenum and the jejunum – are the regions typically affected by CD.

What goes wrong in coeliac disease

The inside of the small intestine is not smooth. The innermost layer that lines it is called the mucosa – the gut lining – and this is characterized by a dense array of small finger-like projections called villi. These provide a large surface area available for the efficient absorption of nutrients through the mucosa.

Gluten is resistant to breakdown. In people without CD, digested gluten fragments are absorbed and dealt with normally, while undigested fragments pass through and out of the body. Any fragments that are absorbed do not appear to pose a problem.

But those with CD aren't so lucky. It seems the lining of the coeliac gut is more 'leaky', allowing gluten fragments through more easily. As people with CD are genetically predisposed to a greater immune sensitivity to gluten, this triggers a response. The reaction is complex, but it is essentially inflammatory and defensive – an attempt by the body to attack the gluten, which it perceives as an invader. The end result is damage to the villi. Over time the villi can become eroded and flattened, sometimes severely, occasionally totally. This is called villous atrophy.

Untreated, this can cause two key problems. First, the ability to produce digestive enzymes is hampered, meaning undigested foods pass through the system to get fermented in the large intestine by bacteria, causing diarrhoea, gastric pain and bloating. Second, damaged villi are less efficient at absorbing nutrients, meaning an increased risk of malnutrition and its complications, such as anaemia, infertility and bone disease.

And, as we know, these are some of the signs of undiagnosed CD.

The changing worldwide picture

While the overall prevalence of CD is thought to be around 1 per cent in the West, there are variations among nations – for example, 2 per cent in Finland and 2.5 per cent in Mexico.

Studies show that the prevalence of CD has increased five-fold, from 0.2 per cent, in the past 40 or 50 years, and that it continues to rise, especially among the elderly. The reasons must be environmental, as the genetic status of the population cannot have changed significantly in such a short period.

The problem of CD in the developing nations is serious. It is a common, often undiagnosed problem in northern India, where wheat is widely consumed (the traditional southern Indian diet is gluten free), and may be the cause of malnutrition in many children.

Some North African rates can be high, though this problem is a little offset by the availability of other traditional grains, such as corn, millet and sorghum, which probably results in a lower expression of the disease. The Saharawi people of southern Algeria demonstrate a CD prevalence of a staggering 7 per cent and are among those most in need of better medical support.

There are few parts of the world where gluten is not consumed – some south Saharan nations, some parts of the Far

East, and New Guinea. Thanks to the general Westernization of the global diet, gluten consumption is likely to continue to rise, and with it the incidence of CD – a particular worry in China, with its high population. Undetected cases will cost economies and health services dearly, and this is likely to remain a huge international challenge in the coming decade.

2
Tests and diagnoses

Coeliac disease can present with many symptoms. If you have digestive and gut problems, a doctor may consider CD, but if these are absent and you have other general and mixed symptoms – which could easily indicate any number of health issues – it may not initially be suspected. Some doctors still see CD as a wasting disease, and will not consider it a possibility when patients are, for example, overweight – even though many are so at diagnosis.

Testing – yes or no?

There are many conditions and situations that may justify testing for CD, and most are specified in guidelines issued by the National Institute for Health and Care Excellence (NICE).

Irregular blood test results

Often, routine blood tests for other medical investigations alert doctors to a need for further tests, including those for CD. Irregular blood cells, low iron or calcium levels, or abnormal liver and kidney function markers, for instance, could indicate a problem. In the absence of any CD symptoms, this is how many cases first reveal themselves, but as there are other reasons for these results, it does depend on your medical practitioner pursuing CD as a possibility along with other suspicions.

Common coeliac symptoms

Aside from the well-known digestive symptoms of diarrhoea, nausea, abdominal pain and so on, other symptoms that should be followed up with testing include faltering growth or failure to thrive (in children), sudden or unexplained weight loss, the unexplained presence of anaemia, and continuing tiredness or fatigue.

Less common coeliac symptoms

Testing should be considered in cases of dental enamel defects, depression or bipolar disorder, epilepsy, certain problems with the bones, unexplained fertility issues and unexplained hair loss.

Irritable bowel syndrome

Irritable bowel syndrome (IBS) is a gut disorder characterized by symptoms such as diarrhoea, constipation, alternating diarrhoea and constipation, bloating, abdominal pain, urgency, incomplete bowel movements and other related complaints.

It is a *functional* gut disorder – a problem with how the intestine works – rather than a *structural* one, in which there would be a physical abnormality detectable by scans, biopsies or examinations.

However, owing to the overlap of symptoms with CD, misdiagnoses of IBS are often made. NICE guidelines for the diagnosis of IBS specify that CD must be ruled out before an IBS diagnosis is made, but if yours was given some years ago, this may not have been undertaken. It is worth talking to your doctor about this, especially if you have been self-managing your IBS for some years. Research suggests CD is four times as common in those who have received an IBS diagnosis than in the rest of the population.

Autoimmune conditions

You should be tested for CD if you have autoimmune thyroid disease or type 1 diabetes.

There are other autoimmune conditions, including Addison's disease, autoimmune liver disease and Sjögren's syndrome, which may be linked to CD. The incidence of CD among patients with these conditions varies, but averages about 5 per cent. It is usually preferable to test, especially if you have more than one autoimmune condition.

Family history

A first-degree relative – child, sibling, parent – with CD means that you too should be tested.

Chromosomal syndromes

CD is five to ten times more common in those with Williams' syndrome, Turner's syndrome or Down's syndrome, and testing should be considered in these cases.

Before testing

Your doctor should explain several points before you, or your child, are tested for CD:

- You should *not* stop consuming gluten or feeding it to your child – or reduce intake.
- The blood tests that you or your child may undergo cannot diagnose CD on their own.
- Positive blood test results will mean that you or your child will probably need an endoscopy and biopsy (see pp. 20–22).
- Negative blood test results will mean that CD is unlikely, but may not rule out it arising in future.

The necessity of diagnosis

Possibly most important to understand before you undergo testing is why the end result – a positive or negative diagnosis – is vital.

A confident positive diagnosis is needed to:

- avoid developmental or growth problems that can result with delays in diagnosing or failure to diagnose CD in children;
- ensure that children can subsequently receive care, treatment and monitoring of their development;
- ensure that you receive continuing care from your doctor and gastroenterologist;
- avoid the increased risks of longer-term complications of undiagnosed CD – which include osteoporosis, decreased fertility, undernutrition and a small increased risk of intestinal cancers;
- confirm that a gluten-free diet (GFD) – a tough undertaking – is indeed necessary;
- qualify you for gluten-free (GF) foods on prescription;

- ensure that you receive help and advice from a dietitian on the GF lifestyle;
- help to alert your first-degree relatives that they have an increased likelihood of CD and should also get tested.

A confident negative diagnosis is needed to:

- help to take your medical advisers a step closer to finding the root of any health problems you're experiencing;
- ensure that there is no reason to restrict your diet unnecessarily;
- help in part to confirm a diagnosis of IBS – which has its own treatments.

Gluten consumption

Undoubtedly the toughest challenge for many is having to continue to eat gluten – or feed it to their child – prior to testing. Blood testing detects antibodies to gluten, which are produced by the immune system of coeliacs. If you stop eating gluten, the body stops producing the antibodies, and the blood tests won't reflect a true picture. It may be particularly hard to consume bread and pasta knowing that they could be harming you.

The recommendation is to eat some gluten in more than one meal every day for at least six weeks before testing. At least 10 grams of gluten a day is thought to be needed – this can be made up of any combination of, for instance, slices of white bread (2–3 grams of gluten each) or wholewheat bread (4–5 grams each), digestive biscuits or rusks (1 gram each), a small serving of pasta (6 grams) or a Weetabix or Shredded Wheat (2 grams each).

Psychologically, it's important to remind yourself how vital it is for you to do this to achieve the ultimate goal of an accurate result, and potentially a life of health and free of symptoms for you or your child. Try to comfort yourself with the knowledge that it will soon be over and you will have an answer. If you find it difficult, speak to your doctor. In some cases, it may be possible to give your child gluten powder hidden in foods that he or she does not associate with feeling poorly.

Blood tests

Routine blood tests, for instance to check for anaemia or liver function, can assist a diagnosis and serve to highlight specific health issues, but dedicated CD tests are key in the diagnostic procedure. These are very good but not 100 per cent accurate, which means they cannot usually diagnose the disease alone.

Which blood tests are offered may vary according to the laboratory conducting the tests, or according to your or your child's medical history and circumstances.

The tissue transglutaminase antibody (tTG or tTGA) test

This looks for antibodies to an enzyme – tissue transglutaminase – produced when the coeliac-affected gut tries to repair itself. It is the first-choice test for adults and children and is easy to perform.

When CD is present in adults, it correctly confirms a positive diagnosis in at least 90 per cent of cases – though false positives are more likely in people with other autoimmune conditions.

When CD is absent, it correctly confirms a negative diagnosis at least 95 per cent of the time.

The test may be less accurate in children.

The endomysial antibody (EMA) test

This looks for antibodies against tissue called endomysium, which joins cells together. It is usually used as an additional test when the results of the tTG test are borderline or uncertain, although it is more expensive and difficult for medical teams to perform.

When CD is present, it correctly confirms a positive diagnosis in 95 per cent of cases. When CD is absent, it correctly confirms a negative diagnosis 99 per cent of the time.

Total immunoglobulin A level

Both the tTG and EMA tests look for classes of antibodies called immunoglobulin A (IgA). However, around 2 per cent of coeliac patients have IgA deficiency – natural low levels of this antibody. If the tTG and EMA tests are negative, an IgA deficiency test may be undertaken. If this is positive, alternative antibodies called immunoglobulin G (IgG) can be used to conduct the tTG and EMA tests instead.

The deamidated gliadin peptide (DGP) antibody test

This tests for antibodies to gluten molecules that have been partially broken down. It may be additionally useful when there is IgA deficiency and/or other blood tests are negative but CD is still strongly suspected.

HLA typing

Virtually all people with CD have one of two genetic tissue types – HLA-DQ2 or HLA-DQ8. Testing for these types, then, can also assist a diagnosis – but usually only in ruling out CD when they are absent.

Home blood tests

Personal testing kits are now available. The Biotech Biocard Celiac Test, for instance, available from pharmacies, is a kit allowing you to take a small sample of your own blood and test it for coeliac IgA antibodies. The results are said to be as accurate as laboratory results, but of course false positives or false negatives are possible. In practice, there is always the danger that a false negative could offer false reassurance. Either outcome should be discussed with your doctor, who will insist on repeating a positive test.

Blood test results

If all blood test results are negative and there is no other clinical reason to suspect CD, a confident negative diagnosis can be made.

If all the blood test results are negative but there remains a strong continuing clinical suspicion of CD – typical symptoms, perhaps teamed with strong family history or other autoimmune illnesses – then a referral for a biopsy of the gut lining may be given.

If any of the key blood test results are positive, you or your child will probably be referred to a gastroenterologist or paediatric gastroenterologist for a biopsy.

However, because positive antibodies to CD can sometimes be temporary in children, there may be occasional circumstances when it is better to take no action and review the situation in six months or a year.

Endoscopy and biopsy

An endoscopy is an internal medical examination using an apparatus called an endoscope, which is passed into the body.

A biopsy is the removal of a little tissue for examination.

An endoscopy and biopsy of the lining of the small intestine to check for coeliac-related damage is usually considered necessary in diagnosing CD. You or your child will have to attend the hospital out-patients department for the procedure, although young children will need to be admitted and given a general anaesthetic. Food and drink must be avoided for a period beforehand, but check with the endoscopy unit in advance. There may be a need to restrict some medications too. Intravenous sedation is available for those nervous of the procedure. Alternatively, a milder anaesthetic can be sprayed at the back of the throat.

A device is placed into your mouth to keep it open. Air will be passed into your body to expand it and allow the endoscopist to see better. The endoscope, which is a long flexible tube, is passed into the mouth, down the throat into the stomach, and then into the duodenum. The end of the endoscope has a light and a camera, and tiny forceps for obtaining small samples of the lining of the gut. Several samples will be taken from different areas, because the damage caused by CD can be patchy.

Typically the procedure will be over in half an hour. It is painless, though if you have anaesthetic spray it will be slightly uncomfortable. The advantage of the spray over sedation is that you can leave the hospital soon after the procedure. If you are sedated, you will need to wait for several hours, be discharged into the care of a friend or relative, and rest afterwards. You should be back to normal within 24 hours, though you will have a slight sore throat.

The tissue samples are sent to a laboratory for microscopic analysis.

In the case of suspected dermatitis herpetiformis (see p. 8), a small biopsy of unaffected skin is taken.

Is a biopsy necessary?

For some years, the biopsy has been considered the 'gold standard' means of confirming a diagnosis, but improvements in blood testing and recognition now mean this view is being increasingly challenged, with some gastroenterologists believing it may sometimes be better not to put a patient through the procedure.

A study from Derby in 2008 found that tTG test results above a certain level could be 100 per cent accurate in diagnosing CD, and that around 50 per cent of tested cases reached this level – meaning that half of patients could avoid a biopsy and be confidently diagnosed on the strength of the blood test alone. Accordingly, some gastroenterologists have begun to adopt this policy when clinical suspicion is strong and tTG readings are high. Diagnosing without a biopsy is also cheaper and does not add burden to health service resources.

A possible advantage of this from a wider perspective is that it could encourage more people to come forward. Some patients with symptoms may be reluctant to present to their doctor and pursue a diagnosis because of fear of a biopsy.

But there *are* advantages for retaining biopsy as a means of diagnosis. It offers certainty – and some feel nobody should have to go on a GFD if there is any possible doubt.

Some also consider it vital to measure the scale of characteristic gut lining erosion as a 'benchmark'. Should the patient continue to experience symptoms after, say, six months on a GFD, a biopsy may sometimes become essential. Without an earlier one for comparison, it would be impossible to determine how much healing has taken place in the meantime.

The results of a biopsy can also serve as a powerful motivator to stick to a GFD: without one, a patient may be less likely to appreciate the seriousness of his or her condition and the internal damage that comes with it, and be more tempted to stray from the diet occasionally.

This issue is much debated among the coeliac community, and recommendations are likely to be modified over time. Indeed, guidelines published in 2013 on the diagnosis of CD in children stated that in some cases, patients with highly positive blood test results and positive HLA typing could be diagnosed confidently without biopsy.

Remember that nobody can force you or your child to have an endoscopy and biopsy, and that each case is unique. Discuss options with your medical team.

Video capsule endoscopy

This involves swallowing a pill that has been fitted internally with a tiny camera that takes images as it moves through the intestine. The photographs are transmitted to a receiver worn on a belt by the patient, and these can be downloaded by doctors to look for inflammation or erosion of the gut's lining.

It is not yet approved as a diagnostic technique for CD, and studies on its effectiveness have found mixed results, albeit some quite positive. That said, it is becoming increasingly available through the health service, and may be useful in those who decline an endoscopy, or for patients whose biopsies are negative despite CD being highly suspected.

Diagnosis

Following testing, there are several possible results.

Blood positive and biopsy positive

This combination of results confirms CD.

Blood positive and biopsy negative

This combination of results could indicate absence of CD and false-positive blood test results. A negative HLA typing test can strengthen the negative diagnosis.

This could also be potential CD, however, which can develop into classical or non-classical CD over time. Your doctor may advise you or your child to stick to a normal, gluten-containing diet and keep the situation under regular review, with perhaps repeat testing in future.

Blood negative and biopsy positive

There are other possible causes of inflammation to the lining – recent gastroenteritis, other gut disorders – and these may need to be excluded. This is especially true of babies and infants, who may have other food sensitivities that cause the damage. Generally, though, this result will be viewed as CD and treated as such.

Blood negative and biopsy negative

CD is currently absent. However, there may be justification to keep monitoring the situation and repeat the blood tests in the future – for instance, in cases of a strong family history or in patients with other autoimmune conditions.

Blood positive and biopsy not performed

If tTG levels are high, and other results suggest CD, this may be enough for some gastroenterologists to diagnose the disease.

Testing negative

A negative test may leave you feeling relieved that you don't have CD but frustrated that you haven't found the cause of any symptoms. Rest assured that you are a step closer, having ruled out one of the possibilities. IBS aside, other conditions may need to be considered.

Non-coeliac gluten sensitivity (NCGS)

There is no recognized blood test for NCGS, and given the uncertainty surrounding it, no standardized method of diagnosis either.

The best solution appears to be in continuing to exclude other possibilities such as WA, and finally undergoing an elimination diet (see p. 120) under the guidance of a dietitian. Assuming symptoms clear, this would conclude with a gluten 'challenge' – preferably 'blind' (so that you are unaware whether what you are given to eat contains gluten or doesn't) – to see whether symptoms then return.

Other food sensitivities

Lactose intolerance is the inability to digest lactose (the sugar in milk), and is caused by a deficiency in lactase, a digestive enzyme. Its symptoms are frothy diarrhoea, abdominal 'gurgling' and bloating. Reliable testing via a hydrogen breath test is available.

Gastrointestinal food allergies may be a possibility, especially in children. These are difficult to diagnose, as reactions can be delayed. Children may need to be investigated for cow's milk protein allergy (CMPA).

Other idiosyncratic food sensitivities may need to be explored using an elimination diet, again with a dietitian.

Inflammatory bowel diseases

Inflammatory bowel diseases, such as Crohn's disease or ulcerative colitis, may need to be considered.

Chronic fatigue syndrome (CFS) and myalgic encephalomyelitis (ME)

These illnesses are characterized by extreme exhaustion, muscle fatigue, problems with concentration, depression and general ill health. There may be digestive symptoms similar to those found in IBS and CD.

Unvalidated testing techniques

There are a number of privately available tests and alternative testing techniques for food sensitivities for which bold claims of their diagnostic capabilities are sometimes made by their manufacturers and the nutritional therapists or practitioners offering them.

None can diagnose CD, and in fairness the manufacturers may well make this clear. However, reference may be made to 'gluten intolerance', 'gluten allergy' or 'wheat sensitivity', among other things. A good rule of thumb is to be very wary of any tests not available through the health service. The tests include:

- electrodermal or Vega testing (available at some high street health stores)
- leukocytotoxicity testing (e.g. NuTron, antigen leukocyte cellular antibody test – ALCAT)
- IgG testing (e.g. YorkTest's FoodScan, CNS's FoodPrint).

There is no evidence to support the use of the first, which is regarded as wholly unscientific. There is insufficient rigorous evidence behind the other two, and most experts in the field believe them to be of no diagnostic use either.

Customers who report improvements after acting on the results of such tests and the recommendations of their practitioners are often merely benefiting from a more nutritious diet. Wheat and dairy are regularly identified as problematic foods, and this constrains consumers to cut out all the calorific or processed food in which these two foods happen to be found – pies, pizzas, hot dogs, burgers, doughnuts, cakes, biscuits and so on. These inevitably have to be replaced by more healthy whole grains, vegetables, fruits, dried fruit and nuts. Often, it is the inclusion of these wholesome foods – not the exclusion of theoretically problematic ones – that is the main reason for improved health.

Some complementary practitioners of applied kinesiology, the Nambudripad allergy elimination technique (NAET), homoeopathy and many other practices may also make claims to be able to diagnose (or treat) food sensitivities. These have no place in modern medicine, and have either failed scientific scrutiny or been discredited by experts. Avoid all when seeking a diagnosis or treatment of any kind.

Self-diagnosis

Self-diagnosis of food sensitivities has become common, is unreliable and is now a potential health concern.

To some extent, it has been popularized by celebrities and fad-diet enthusiasts who have blamed wheat, gluten, dairy, sugar, soya and other foods for various Western ills. The encouragement, often via social media, of people who believe they have successfully self-diagnosed is also contributing to the problem.

Many patients take to 'Dr Google' and either self-diagnose or place themselves on experimental, limited diets, which could affect their nutritional status, all on the basis of questionable information found online.

Feeling better following the exclusion of a food or food component does not imply a sensitivity to it, as there could be several reasons for health improvement (other components of the excluded foods, benefits derived from replacement foods, psychological improvements, etc.).

It can be dangerous to self-diagnose because it is easy to misinterpret symptoms, and this may mean serious conditions are missed. Avoiding gluten may mean future coeliac blood tests are unreliable and, ironically, avoiding dairy may eventually lead to lactose intolerance that may not have existed beforehand, as the body scales down its production of the enzyme lactase when dairy is avoided.

An Australian survey published in 2014 found that almost three-quarters of patients who self-diagnosed NCGS did not satisfy its criteria. Many had not had CD excluded, and some were experiencing symptoms despite following a GFD.

It is understandable that individuals who have been investigated unsuccessfully for any number of possible diseases or conditions should eventually self-diagnose a food sensitivity as a last resort, but in this exceptional instance it is strongly advised you only do so with the knowledge of your doctor and under the care of a dietitian – especially if you are restricting several foods.

3
Food sense: labelling and shopping

The key aspect of successful, long-term management of coeliac disease is a diet free from gluten. When you are diagnosed you should be referred to a dietitian – or a paediatric dietitian in the case of a child. However, there may be a delay before your first consultation, so you will need to try to get to grips with the basics of the gluten-free diet (GFD) right away.

The gluten-free diet

A GFD is a diet that *excludes* the following gluten-containing grains:

- wheat
- barley
- rye.

It also excludes:

- all varieties of wheat (e.g. durum, einkorn, emmer, Kamut® or khorosan, spelt)
- all forms of wheat (e.g. bran, bulgur, couscous, freekeh, rusk, semolina, wheat protein, wheat starch, wheatgerm)
- hybrids of the gluten grains, such as triticale (a wheat–rye hybrid), some oats and oat products (but see p. 37).

So the GFD must exclude all products containing the grains listed above and all products containing ingredients derived from them – with few exceptions (see p. 31 and p. 38). It therefore excludes, for example, ordinary breads, pastas, cakes, biscuits, many cereals, and many flour-containing products and pre-prepared meals.

It *includes* all fruit, vegetables, nuts, seeds, non-gluten grains, meats, fish, natural dairy products and eggs, and products and ingredients derived only from these foods.

The wheat problem

Although there are several grains you need to avoid, it is wheat that you'll encounter most regularly. It is widespread in the Western diet, partly because flour-based products such as breads and pastas are staples, and partly because of wheat's additional role as a stabilizer, thickener or 'filler' in processed foods. It may be used to 'dust' products and prevent them clumping together, and can turn up in surprising places. Wheat-based or wheat-containing products may include:

- most flours, breads and baked products – both sweet and savoury
- many cereals
- most pastas, some noodles
- processed meat and fish products – burgers, pies, sausages, pâtés and battered products such as fish fingers
- processed vegetarian products – battered vegetables, pâtés, some tinned soups, some plant milks
- some processed dairy products, such as cheese spreads, thickened milks and creams
- confectionery, including chocolate bars, cereal bars, sweets, chewing gum and liquorice
- miscellaneous products such as stock cubes, gravy granules, condiments and blended seasonings.

Labelling, ingredients – and allergens

Because so many foods – and some drinks – may contain gluten, you will need to master the skill of label reading. Labels on prepacked products can carry vast amounts of information, much of which many people ignore or misunderstand. As a coeliac, you cannot afford to do either.

Some information is optional; some is required by law.

Optional information includes serving suggestions, recipes and certain nutritional information (such as vitamin and mineral content, in particular circumstances).

Compulsory information includes the food's name, its weight or volume, its use-by or best-before date and contact details of the manufacturers – although there are occasional exceptions. Key nutritional information is required on all products – namely, energy (both in kJ and kcals) and the quantities of fat, saturates, carbohydrates, sugars, protein and salt present.

However, the most useful information is the list of ingredients, which is compulsory on all products with the exception of single-ingredient products (such as a carton of milk or a packet of barley) and most alcoholic beverages. It presents all ingredients used deliberately in the product's manufacture, in descending order of weight.

The list obviously includes all whole foods. These include names of vegetables, fruits, grains and nuts, for instance. It also includes ingredients derived from whole foods, and whose sources may not be provided or obvious (e.g. 'vinegar' or 'sugar').

Further, the list also may include general collective terms, the details of which may not be supplied or clear either (e.g. 'flavourings' or 'spices') and of course any additives and colourings.

And then there are compound ingredients, which may themselves have their own ingredients, sometimes given in brackets (e.g. 'salami [contains pork, salt, spices, seasonings]').

According to European legislation, certain foods must *always* be named on the ingredients list – not only when they are present as whole foods, but also when they are the source of an ingredient or are found in a compound ingredient. (There are exemptions: see p. 31.)

There are 14 such foods or food groups, and they are often described as the main or declarable food allergens. Although CD is not a food allergy, gluten-containing cereals *are* a food allergen group, and for clarity and simplicity should be considered food allergens even in a coeliac context.

The 14 have been chosen because they are the most commonly and dangerously problematic ones for people who react to foods. The full list is:

- celery (and celeriac)
- cereal grains containing gluten – barley, oats, rye and all types of wheat (including common, durum, khorosan and spelt wheats), or their hybrids
- crustaceans (e.g. crab, lobster, prawn)
- eggs
- fish
- lupin
- milk (including milk sugar, or lactose)
- molluscs (e.g. mussel, snail, squid)
- mustard
- tree nuts (namely almonds, hazelnuts, Brazil nuts, cashews, pistachios, macadamia nuts, walnuts and pecans)
- peanuts
- sesame seeds
- soya beans
- sulphur dioxide and sulphites.

To give an example of a food being used to manufacture an ingredient, let's take 'sugar'. The source of 'sugar' as an ingredient does not need to be specified as 'cane sugar' or 'beet sugar', because neither cane nor beet is on the list of 14. However, the source of malt vinegar – barley – must be stated.

Emphasizing of allergens

Legislation that came into full effect in December 2014 specified that the 14 key allergens or allergen groups should be emphasized in lists of ingredients when they are present, in order to make them stand out clearly.

Most manufacturers use **bold** to emphasize these allergens, but some use <u>underlining</u>, *italics*, CAPITALS, a different font colour, a different background colour or a combination of these.

With regard to the gluten grains, if the grain features in the ingredient's name, only the grain should be emphasized: e.g. '**wheat** flour' (or '<u>wheat</u> flour' or '*wheat* flour', etc.).

If the ingredient's name partly consists of the grain, either the whole word should be emphasized or just the grain: e.g. '**oatmeal** flour' or '**oat**meal flour'.

Where the name of the grain does not feature in the ingredient's name, it should be supplied and emphasized alongside: e.g. 'couscous (**wheat**)'.

The addition of the word 'gluten' is optional, but if used it will *not* be emphasized: e.g. either '**rye** flour (gluten)' or '**rye** flour' may be used.

The word 'gluten' is compulsory *only* when gluten itself is the ingredient. Again, the source grain must be given and emphasized – *not* the word 'gluten': e.g. 'gluten (**barley**)' or '**barley** gluten'.

Exemptions

Derivatives of the 14 allergens that have undergone so much processing or refining that they are no longer considered a risk to consumers are exempt from the legislation. As far as the gluten-containing cereals are concerned, these exemptions are:

- wheat-based or barley-based glucose syrups, including dextrose
- wheat-based maltodextrins
- cereals used for distillates and spirits in alcoholic beverages.

These are all considered safe for coeliacs and those with wheat or barley allergy, and manufacturers do *not* need to declare the source grain. If they do choose to declare the cereal, they do *not* need to emphasize it.

In practice, this may mean several possible representations of the same ingredient, e.g.:

- 'glucose syrup'
- 'wheat glucose syrup'
- '**wheat** glucose syrup'.

The third example is rarely used as it can be misleading, but if you see it, or the other options, in reference to an exempt ingredient, it does *not* mean you need to avoid the product – unless there are other ingredients that are unsafe, of course.

Allergy advice statements

Although it is not a legal requirement, many food manufacturers include an additional allergy advice statement on products.

Such statements are intended to direct consumers towards the list of ingredients and explain the method used for emphasizing allergens. For example:

> 'Allergy advice: for allergens, including cereals containing gluten, see ingredients in bold'.

Prior to December 2014, manufacturers could make 'contains' statements within their voluntary allergy advice statements, reiterating the presence of allergens already mentioned in the ingredients. This repetition is no longer permitted, so you will *not* see a 'contains wheat' statement, for example, on a product which carries a list of ingredients (you may see such a statement on a single-ingredient product with no list of ingredients, such as a packet of couscous grains, or on certain alcoholic beverages – see p. 40). Information about allergens present is now located in one place only: the ingredients list.

Allergy advice statements are optional, so if one is absent from a product do not assume the product is either safe or unsafe. Check ingredients.

'May contain' and other allergen warnings

Examples of so-called advisory labelling include 'may contain traces of gluten', 'made in a factory which also handles wheat' or 'may not be suitable for coeliacs'.

Such labelling may be used by manufacturers for two reasons: to warn the public that wheat (or other allergens, often nuts), although not intentionally added, might have accidentally contaminated a product or one or more of its ingredients somewhere along the harvesting, transporting or manufacturing line; and also to disclaim any liability should a customer suffer a reaction.

Manufacturers are advised that such labelling should be used only when, following a thorough risk assessment, they believe there is a real risk of cross-contamination.

Coeliac UK says that it can contact manufacturers to talk through the risk, and it does sometimes list such products in its annual handbook, the *Food and Drink Guide* (see p. 41) following discussions with the manufacturers about the production facility and measures to minimize cross-contamination. If you're concerned, contact the charity or the manufacturer for information about suitability. It may well be that the product is safe.

Labels for gluten-free products and Codex standards

So the *presence* of gluten and gluten-containing cereals is conveyed on labels via the ingredients list, but how is their *absence* communicated to consumers?

Since 2012, there have been strict standards in place in the EU for the use of terms on products relating to gluten content. These are called the Codex standards for gluten, named after an international body, the Codex Alimentarius Commission, created over 50 years ago to set up food guidelines.

'Gluten free'

In practice, it is neither possible for manufacturers to achieve, nor possible for scientists to measure, a zero level of gluten in products.

Any products whose ingredients have been processed to remove gluten will have residual traces of it – as will some other foods that are naturally free of gluten but that may pick up trace contamination during production processes.

Research suggests that coeliacs can tolerate foods containing up to 20 parts of gluten per million (20 ppm). This is equivalent to 0.002 per cent or to 20 mg per kg.

Manufacturers can make a 'gluten free' claim for a product if they can demonstrate it meets this standard – i.e. that it contains between 0 and 20 ppm of gluten.

If manufacturers submit their products for laboratory testing and purchase the rights to use Coeliac UK's Crossed Grain trade mark, which depicts a line through an ear of wheat (see Figure 3.1), they can reproduce that symbol on their products to denote they meet the 'gluten free' standard. Some producers and supermarkets use their own, similar logos.

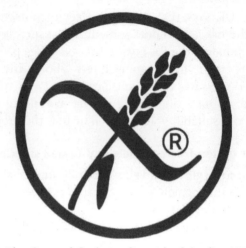

Figure 3.1 The Crossed Grain trade mark of Coeliac UK

Used with permission. Registered trade mark to Coeliac UK

'Very low gluten'

Products containing between 20 and 100 parts of gluten per million (20–100 ppm) can be labelled 'very low gluten' according to the standards. This is more common on products available in northern Europe, and applies only to foods whose cereal ingredients have been processed to remove gluten – not 'normal' foods that happen to fall within the 20–100 ppm range, for which a 'very low gluten' claim cannot be made.

Gluten at these levels may cause problems for some coeliacs, so it is not intended that foods in this category be consumed in large amounts, but they are probably safe at least occasionally for many.

'Suitable for coeliacs' and 'suitable for people intolerant to gluten'

These optional terms may be used, but only to supplement and accompany either a 'gluten free' or 'very low gluten' claim. Alternative phrasing – e.g. 'specifically formulated for coeliacs' – may be seen.

'No gluten-containing ingredients'

Until a few years ago, this statement was occasionally seen on foods, but in 2016 the Food Standards Agency (FSA) pointed out that it was not compliant with labelling law which held that the absence or reduced presence of gluten could only be conveyed through the statements 'gluten free' or 'very low gluten'. It was explicitly banned in 2018, so it (and similar variants) should no longer be seen on individual products.

'Wheat free'

The term 'wheat free' is not defined under Codex standards, and a product bearing it may not be gluten free, since it could contain rye or barley, for example. Furthermore, be aware that 'wheat free' claims are occasionally used inappropriately on products containing spelt, which is a form of wheat.

Understanding 'gluten free'

The term 'gluten free' is enshrined in law and defined to mean something different from what, intuitively, one might suppose it means. It does *not* mean zero gluten. It means 0–20 ppm of gluten.

Think of 'gluten free' as an *absolute* term: a food either is or is not 'gluten free'. There are no degrees of 'gluten free' – a food testing at 8 ppm levels is equally 'gluten free' to one testing at 15 ppm – and no qualification of the term is permitted on labelling.

Manufacturers are therefore only allowed to use those expressions described on pp. 33–34 and *not* such terms as '100 per cent gluten free', 'virtually gluten free' or 'naturally gluten free'. Non-standard claims such as 'reduced gluten content' and 'gluten friendly' are disallowed, and strictly even 'free from gluten' is not permitted either, although it is commonly seen.

The term is simply 'gluten free' – and it is a very powerful claim. Unless you have another sensitivity that requires you to check labelling, a 'gluten free' claim for a product tells you it is safe.

Labelling stumbling blocks

Food labelling rules are complicated, but be assured that most products will not be too difficult to judge for safety, especially as you become more skilled.

Products with certain ingredients can be trickier to gauge for suitability, though, and can confuse many coeliacs, especially those newly diagnosed.

Barley malt – and its derivatives

Malt refers to cereal grains, usually barley, that have been sprouted and then heated and dried. Barley malt or malted barley is *not* suitable for coeliacs.

The sugar-rich syrup derived from malted grains is called malt extract and its flavouring is malt flavouring. Barley malt extract and barley malt flavouring each contain small amounts of gluten. They are used as flavour enhancers, commonly in breakfast cereals. However, in some cereals they are used in such small amounts that the overall gluten levels of the products are below 20 ppm, and are therefore GF. Coeliac UK includes such cereals in its *Food and Drink Guide*. (Some specialist 'free from' producers make breakfast cereals such as corn flakes using rice malt or without malt at all.)

Some products, such as malted drinks and malt beer, use high levels of malt products and these are *not* safe.

Unless you see a 'gluten free' statement, it may not be clear whether a product containing barley malt extract or flavouring is suitable for you. In this case, it is worth checking in the *Food and Drink Guide*, or calling the manufacturer, as it may well be safe.

Malt vinegar is made from barley malt, which is fermented twice – first to produce a kind of ale, and then to convert it to vinegar. It is sold in bottles, and as an ingredient is used in pickles, condiments and sauces. Coeliac UK considers it GF – but some US coeliac bodies disagree, because it is not distilled. Indeed, bottled malt vinegar brands often state they contain gluten. This is a regular subject of debate and concern among coeliacs, and many feel, because all other pure vinegars (e.g. cider, balsamic, red wine, distilled, spirit) are unanimously agreed to be GF, that it is more sensible to choose alternatives instead. When barley malt vinegar is used as an ingredient in a product making a GF claim, the product will be safe, as it will have tested at under 20 ppm. Those choosing not to exclude barley malt vinegar should be reassured that their trace consumption of gluten through it is likely to be extremely low, as it is normally used in such small quantities.

All barley malt derivatives must declare their source on labelling. Remember that in these cases the word 'barley' will be emphasized in lists of ingredients, even if the product itself is GF:

e.g. '**barley** malt flavouring' or 'malt vinegar (**barley**)'. This is to alert people with barley allergy.

Malt whisky, which is distilled, is safe.

Oats

For the purposes of allergy-labelling legislation, oats are considered gluten-containing cereals. However, evidence suggests that the 'gluten' protein in oats (called avenin) is not toxic to most people with CD at everyday levels (but see p. 53).

Reactions to oats are more likely to be due to contamination from wheat flour – and hence wheat gluten – occurring at some point during harvesting, milling or transportation. Some manufacturers of oats will make an allergy advice statement – e.g. 'produced in a factory also handling wheat' – telling you they could be contaminated.

Uncontaminated oats manufactured or processed under strict conditions can make a 'gluten free' claim if they meet Codex standards. Coeliac UK lists such oats and oat-containing cereals in its *Food and Drink Guide*.

Because single-ingredient products don't need to carry an ingredient listing, a packet of oats need not bear any additional information other than its name. Take care with terms such as 'pure oats' or '100 per cent oats' – this does *not* necessarily mean the oats are uncontaminated or GF.

Any products that include oats as an ingredient and carrying a 'gluten free' claim must use oats that meet the Codex standard too.

The word 'oat' or 'oats' should be emphasized in a list of ingredients, even when the products and the oats used are GF. This is to alert people with oat allergy, as well as those coeliacs who react to them.

Codex wheat starch

Ordinary wheat starch is not GF as it has enough residual gluten to cause problems for coeliacs, but there is a special type of wheat starch that is GF, which is permitted for use in foods labelled 'gluten free' or 'very low gluten'. It is almost exclusively found in some prescription foods (see p. 50) that comply with Codex standards.

The starch is called Codex wheat starch – or just 'Codex' among coeliacs. The starch is made through a repeated rinsing process, using only water, and it is suitable for use in products such as breads and flour mixes, offering good taste and baking qualities and a lighter texture.

It will be specified in the ingredients list, and the word 'wheat' will be emphasized, e.g. 'gluten-free **wheat** starch'.

Emphasized gluten grains on safe products

There are a number of cases (see pp. 36–8) where you may see gluten-containing cereals emphasized in lists of ingredients on products that may in fact be GF – and therefore suitable for you.

Bear in mind that food allergen labelling is intended not only for those with CD, but for those with food allergies, food intolerances and other dietary restrictions too.

People with a barley allergy may react to the trace levels of protein in barley malt extract, barley malt vinegar or barley malt flavouring in products containing them that may be safe for coeliacs. Emphasizing the word 'barley' in these cases is a warning to them, not necessarily to those with CD.

Similarly, those with wheat allergy will probably need to avoid Codex wheat starch, and consumers who are sensitive to oats – some coeliacs included – need to be warned about their presence via emphasis, even when they are GF.

Remember: when you come across such ingredients always check other emphasized ingredients – and any allergy advice statement too, where an absence of any reference to 'cereals containing gluten' should be reassuring.

Manufacturers are advised *not* to use a 'may contain gluten' advisory statement on a product that includes a gluten-containing ingredient – such as barley malt extract – but that is able to meet an overall GF standard, because this could be misleading.

Commonly confused ingredients

The derivation and source of certain ingredients regularly cause concern among coeliacs, but remember that unless it is a safe exemption (p. 31), any ingredient derived from a gluten-containing cereal must declare and emphasize the cereal in the ingredients list.

Hydrolysed vegetable protein (HVP) can be derived from a number of sources, including gluten containing grains. If so, it may appear as 'hydrolysed **wheat** protein' or 'hydrolysed vegetable protein (**wheat**)'. HVP that doesn't declare a source will be derived from a food not on the list of 14 allergens, probably corn, and will be safe.

Similarly, ingredients such as 'modified starch', 'cellulose' and 'fibre' will declare the source if it is a gluten grain. If no grain is mentioned, the source will be corn, rice or other foods.

Textured vegetable protein (TVP) is normally from soya; as this is an allergen, it should be declared. It is GF.

Maltitol and isomalt, despite their names, are unrelated to barley malt and are confirmed safe by Coeliac UK.

Spelt

Most wheat used in the food industry is either 'common' wheat (in bakery) or 'durum' wheat (in pasta).

Other wheats, especially spelt, are often mistakenly believed to be GF grains. This error crops up regularly on the internet and occasionally in the media, and even some food outlets have been known to get it wrong.

To reinforce the wheaten status of these less common grains, an emphasized reference to wheat must be made in an ingredients list when one is used in a product, e.g. 'spelt (**wheat**)' or 'khorosan **wheat** flour'.

Food shopping

Shopping for a GFD can be frustrating and time-consuming, but the situation is improving, with increased 'coeliac awareness' of manufacturers, improved labelling and the wider availability of GF foods.

Just been diagnosed? Plan carefully for your first major shop, and go when you have time to devote to it, perhaps during a quiet period when you won't feel stressed. Draw up a list: if you forget to buy a specialist GF product at a major supermarket, you may not be able to find it at your local store. It is important to understand labelling basics before you set off. If you do the bulk of your shopping at the supermarket you can continue to do so: it's unlikely you'll have to change your routine drastically.

The ingredients for everyday GF meals – baked potatoes and beans, rice dishes, 'meat and two veg', homemade vegetable soups – will probably be on your menu, but don't be afraid to try new naturally GF foods.

Been diagnosed a while? Perhaps you're stuck in a rut of eating the same old meals, and haven't evaluated your diet for some time? Again, consider investing more time at your supermarket and other, smaller food stores. You may be surprised at the quantity of alternative and GF food now available.

Alcoholic beverages

Alcoholic drinks of greater than 1.2 per cent strength are subject to less strict labelling regulations, and an ingredients list is optional. However, any key food allergens, including gluten-containing grains, must be declared in one of three possible ways:

- in the product's name (e.g. 'Wheat Ale');
- within a list of ingredients (where it should be emphasized, in the same way as any other product);
- via an allergy advice statement (where it might not be emphasized, e.g. 'Contains: barley').

In practice, this will usually apply only to beers, given that spirits such as whisky distilled from gluten-containing cereals – which fall under the exemptions (see p. 31) – are GF.

Ordinary beers are off-limits to coeliacs, but specialist GF beers are now available. Some of these are made from sorghum or millet, for example, but most are from barley. In the latter cases, brewers add specialist enzymes to the beers during production to break down the gluten proteins to a level that coeliacs can tolerate. Like the situation with barley malt vinegar (see p. 36), this is an active area of discussion within the coeliac community, mainly because of the testing methods employed to measure trace gluten in beer, which some believe may not be sufficiently accurate. Many coeliacs consume so-called gluten reduced and enzyme-treated beers without apparent problem, but others avoid them. Such a beer can easily be identified as by law its label must state that it contains the gluten containing cereal (usually barley, but very occasionally wheat and/or oats too).

For alcoholic drinks weaker than 1.2 per cent, standard labelling rules apply. Low-alcohol and alcohol-free GF beers are starting to become available.

Food directories

Coeliac UK's annual *Food and Drink Guide* lists around 10,000 safe products and is an invaluable guide. Updated every January, it is divided into sections: prescription products, 'free from' products, everyday products and supermarket own-brand products. Monthly updates are made available via various means.

It is not exhaustive. Not all companies are willing or able to provide the information required by the charity – even those whose products carry confirmation that they are suitable for coeliacs. Therefore, products not listed in the *Food and Drink Guide* may well be safe. It is important to read labels and, if necessary, ring the manufacturers' helplines for advice. Many manufacturers and smaller supermarkets whose products do not appear in the *Food and Drink Guide* can send you lists of safe foods.

The Coeliac Society of Ireland produces the *Food List*, the Irish equivalent of the *Food and Drink Guide*.

'Free from' foods

So-called 'free from' foods are foods manufactured to be free from one or more of the key food allergens that would normally be expected to be present in the food. Usually, this means gluten free and dairy free – but egg-free and nut-free foods are increasingly popular too.

It is these foods on which you're most likely to find the term 'gluten free', and many of them feature in the *Food and Drink*

Guide. Many supermarkets also have lists of their own-brand 'free from' foods, which they can send you by email.

The 'free from' sector boomed during the first decade of this century, with huge year-on-year growth, and many manufacturers now specialize in these ranges. Most supermarkets and health-food stores stock a range of such products, and in larger branches you'll find 'free from' sections or aisles devoted to foods for restricted diets, including many own-brand foods. Bear in mind, however, that most but *not* all foods in 'free from' sections will be GF. Always check labels. Some milk-free and egg-free products, marketed as vegan products and stocked in 'free from' sections, can and do contain wheat and other gluten-containing cereals. 'Free from' does *not* always necessarily mean 'gluten free'.

It hasn't always been like this. As recently as the early part of the millennium, the selection was pretty grim for coeliacs, with poor-quality breads, which were heavy and grey-tinged and easily fell apart – never mind the odd taste. Now, some of the breads are light, tasty and barely discernible from standard loaves. Then there's the sheer variety: baguettes, ciabattas, rolls, pittas, white, brown, stoneground, multi-grain, wraps, pizza bases . . . And it's not just breads: there are abundant GF noodles, pastas, pastries, pies, fish fingers, sausage rolls, quiches, Scotch eggs – and much more.

Growth is predicted to ease off, but innovation and continued demand is likely to keep the market buoyant, as CD diagnoses and interest in the GF lifestyle rise and greater competition drives further improvement. New technologies (improved methods for 'deglutenizing', for instance) and the bolder use of more exotic GF grains (such as teff and quinoa) hold promise for coeliac gourmets.

Drawbacks

There are downsides to 'free from' foods, though.

First, they can be dearer, because of the cost of allergen testing and specialist ingredients, and the difficulty of manufacture, among other reasons.

Second, they're not always the healthiest of products. Some can be higher in fat and sugar, and may require a host of additives. They're terrific in helping you make the transition to the GFD after diagnosis when everything is confusing and you may be fearful of what you can or can't eat, but it's probably wise not to come to rely on them too much in the long term.

Third, manufacturers are occasionally guilty of making an inappropriate virtue of their 'free from' status. Products proclaiming 'no baddies' or 'allergy friendly' should be treated with the same critical eye as any other food you're evaluating. Table 3.1 gives a checklist of safe foods, foods that must be checked and foods that are not GF.

Other foods

Plenty of foods not specifically aimed at coeliacs will of course be suitable. Some may not make a gluten-specific claim because the manufacturers can't afford or do not wish to pay for rigorous testing or a licence to use the Crossed Grain trade mark.

Thousands of such foods are listed in Section 2 of the *Food and Drink Guide*.

This table is intended as a guide to GF and non-GF foods – and foods that usually need to be checked. Never use it in place of careful reading of the label, because occasional exceptions arise.

Table 3.1 Food checklist

	Gluten free	Must be checked	Not gluten free
Grains, flours, starches	Rice, corn and maize, millet, buckwheat, quinoa, sorghum, amaranth, teff. Flours and starches made from these grains – such as polenta (cornmeal) – from soya, chickpeas (gram), lentils and chestnut, and from tapioca (cassava), potatoes and other root vegetables (but see right). GF oats. Codex wheat starch.	Some flours produced from gluten-free grains (see left) may be contaminated if milled alongside gluten-containing grains. Oats and oat products	Wheat (including wheatgerm, bran, bulgur, durum, semolina, couscous, spelt, kamut), rye, barley, triticale, contaminated oats. All ordinary flours and flours made from the above grains.

(Continued)

Table 3.1 (*Continued*)

	Gluten free	Must be checked	Not gluten free
Pasta and noodles	Pastas and noodles from the above grains and flours, including pure corn pasta and rice or buckwheat noodles. Specialist GF pastas.	Some buckwheat noodles or spaghetti may contain wheat	Italian pastas and wheat noodles.
Bakery products	Baked goods made from above grains and flours. GF bread, biscuits and cakes	Macaroons. Baking powder. Corn tortilla wraps	All ordinary breads, pizzas, biscuits and cakes.
Breakfast cereals	GF cereals and muesli mix. GF oats	Corn flakes, rice pops and other malted cereals (see p. 36). Oats and oat mueslis. All other cereals not labelled GF and not clearly wheat-based	All wheat-based cereals (Shredded Wheat, bran flakes).
Meat and fish	All fresh, frozen, smoked and cured pure meats. All fish and shellfish. Pure tinned fish	Meat and fish pâtés and pastes. Sausages, smoked sausage and salamis. Burgers. Prepared meat and fish dishes and ready meals. Tinned meats. Sushi. Crabsticks and seafood sticks. Suet	Meat and fish products in batter or breadcrumbs. Meat and fish pies and pasties. Fishcakes and fish fingers. Taramasalata.
Vegetables, fruit and nuts	All vegetables and fruit. Vegetable oils and fats. All nuts and seeds and their oils, such as peanut, hazelnut, sesame, sunflower, hemp. Pure ground almonds	Prepared salads. Ready-made potato products (e.g. instant mash, waffles, chips). Tinned soups and vegetables. Fruit fillings. Roasted nuts and seed or trail mixes	Breaded vegetables and tempura. Vegetarian pâtés.

	Gluten free	Must be checked	Not gluten free
Dairy products and eggs	Milk, yoghurt, cream, butter, unprocessed cheese. Eggs	Thickened milks and creams. Processed, spreadable or cream cheeses. Coffee whiteners	Scotch eggs
Vegetarian and vegan foods	Plain tofu and bean curd. Quorn. Hummus	Veggie burgers. Soya-based products. Ready-made vegetarian products. Vegetarian proteins. Flavoured or marinated tofu. Vegetable and nut milks (e.g. soya, hazelnut milk). Soya desserts. Vegetable suet	Most oat milk
Drinks	Fruit and vegetable juices. Pure herbal teas. Teas, coffees. Wine, spirits, cider, GF beers	Drinking chocolate. Cloudy drinks. Cola drinks. Coffee substitutes	Ordinary beers, ales and lagers. Malted drinks. Barley waters.
Snacks	Rice cakes and crackers. Natural popcorn	Crisps and related savoury snacks. Tortilla chips	Pretzels
Spreads	Honey, jam, marmalade, sugar syrups (treacle, molasses)	Nut butters. Lemon curd. Yeast spreads	—
Sauces and seasonings	Vinegar (including malt). Herbs, pure spices, garlic, salt and pepper	Stock and stock cubes, bouillon. Packet sauces, jarred sauces. Relishes, mustard products, marinades. Mayonnaise and salad cream. Blended seasonings. Curry powder, mix and sauce. Japanese soy sauce. Worcestershire sauce	Chinese soy sauce

(Continued)

Table 3.1 (*Continued*)

	Gluten free	Must be checked	Not gluten free
Sweets and desserts	Jellies. Sweeteners. Sugar	Meringue. Chocolate and chocolate products. Confectionery. Ice creams. Ready-made desserts. Liquorice. Custard powders. Blancmanges. Mincemeat	Semolina puddings. Ice cream cones and wafers.

Product recalls and food alerts

Mistakes can occur in food manufacturing. Products can be misla-belled, or get contaminated with food allergens, and find their way on to the shelf before the error is detected. When noticed, though, the food industry leaps into action, and there are several ways in which messages will be conveyed to consumers.

Coeliac UK's website carries all product recalls issued that are of concern to coeliacs. The Food Standards Agency issues food alerts, including allergen alerts. Click to <www.food.gov.uk/enforcement/alerts>, where you can register to receive them.

If you come to rely on certain companies' products, subscribe to their mailing lists, so they can reach you in the event of a relevant food alert.

Read any conspicuous 'product recall' signs in supermarkets; these may be located where the products are stocked.

Non-prepacked food

Since December 2014, businesses selling non-prepacked food sold loose at bakeries, takeaways, butchers and deli counters, for example, have had to provide information on which of the 14 declarable allergens they contain.

This can be provided via a chalkboard or information pack, for example. It can also be supplied orally via a member of staff, though if this is the case it must be signposted that customers should ask for it, and the information supplied in this way should be consistent and verifiable, if challenged.

Food businesses are not permitted to plead ignorance about the allergens their foods contain, and neither can they declare that all their products 'may contain' the 14 key allergens. They will be legally obliged to provide accurate information.

Gluten-related claims can be made for loose foods, but the same standards as for prepacked foods apply.

Note that there is no obligation to provide a full list of ingredients for non-prepacked foods – though many will do so.

'Prepacked for direct sale' food

In the summer of 2019, a new law was agreed mandating that food prepared on-site and prepacked for direct sale at the same premises should carry full ingredient labelling. So-called Natasha's Law was named after Natasha Ednan-Laperouse, a teenage girl who died in 2016 after eating an unlabelled wrap containing sesame, to which she was allergic. The food industry has until the summer of 2021 to comply with this regulation, which will mainly effect foods such as sandwiches and salads. The law will not apply to foods sold 'loose', unpackaged, or only prepared and wrapped at the customer's order and request. These foods are considered non-prepacked food.

International foods

Although wheat is the dominant grain and source of starchy carbohydrate in Western society and cuisine, it isn't in many overseas food cultures. Markets, stores and delicatessens devoted to international cuisines can offer an eye-opening array of foods for you to explore, albeit perhaps when you are feeling more adventurous and settled into GF life. Look out for Japanese soba (buckwheat) noodles, Mexican mesquite flour, Korean sweet potato vermicelli, Chinese bean curd noodles, Vietnamese tapioca sticks, and more.

Shopping online

The major supermarkets now act as internet retailers too and their sites allow you either to tick a box in order to filter out non-'free from' foods and/or specify GF, or to enter 'gluten' in a search field, which should reveal available GF foods. Nutritional information, ingredients and allergens are provided.

The advantages of shopping this way are clear: it's time-saving, you can browse at leisure at all hours and you can buy long-lasting and heavy food products in bulk and have them delivered.

Weighed against this must be delivery costs, and perhaps having to plan ahead what you want to eat over coming weeks. It's also not quite the same as browsing and examining a product close up – unless you've bought the product before, it's not always easy to know what you're getting.

Online 'free from' retailers, specializing in products for all those on restricted diets, are thriving. Even internet behemoth Amazon stocks a huge range, but others are listed in 'Useful addresses'. Check deliveries carefully when they arrive, though, as mistakes can happen.

Online 'cottage' industries

There has been growth too in the number of small, often home-based or family-run businesses, trading mainly online.

Many are owned and staffed by coeliacs, who understand the needs of those on the GFD well. Quality is usually high. Products are often hand-made, using mostly natural and sometimes locally sourced ingredients, low in additives. Some offer personal and 'bespoke' services – for instance, cakes for special celebrations, incorporating other dietary needs too.

Many are so small-scale, though, that they may not be able to afford tests needed to demonstrate they meet Codex standards, even if the ingredients they use do meet them and they maintain a working environment free from gluten. Word of mouth and online chat forums are a good way to source recommendations.

4

Food sense: eating and dining out

In Chapter 3 we learned about the gluten-free diet, food labelling and food ingredients, and the variety of specialist 'free from' foods available. That was the 'food sense' *theory*.

Now comes the *practice* – actually putting that knowledge of safe foods to work on your eating and dining lifestyle and habits. And there's one person who can help you in this regard more than anyone else.

Your dietitian

When you are diagnosed with coeliac disease you should be referred to a registered dietitian – a trained and qualified professional who can help to translate the science of nutrition into personalized practical dietary advice and guidance. Dietitians are understanding and supportive, and many specialize in restricted diets or food sensitivities. A child with CD will see a paediatric dietitian.

It is important you see your dietitian regularly and build up a strong relationship because evidence shows that those regularly in touch with their dietitians stick more rigidly and healthily to the GFD in the long term and have more satisfactory health outcomes.

Your first appointment

In the days leading up to your first appointment, keep a one-week food diary of everything you, or your child, eat and drink, and when. Your dietitian will want to know about your diet in order to help best plan replacement foods and meals that are nutritionally adequate, and a diary will give a more accurate reflection as your memory can be unreliable.

Take a list of questions with you. Take notepaper and don't be embarrassed to write down answers. Your dietitian will give you lots of information, but without taking notes you will not remember it all, although she (most dietitians are women) will supply you with leaflets.

During the appointment your dietitian will go through a number of key issues with you:

- what gluten and CD are and how both affect the body;
- gluten-containing foods, safe foods, food labelling, food shopping and the implications of the GFD;
- gluten-free products available on prescription (see below), the companies that produce them, and perhaps some samples or vouchers;
- aspects of health – weight, symptoms, any improvements or problems since diagnosis, exercise, smoking, alcohol intake, etc.;
- any dietary restrictions – vegetarian, co-existing food allergies;
- cooking and eating out (see pp. 54–65).

One of your dietitian's key aims will be to impress upon you the value of the GFD and how quickly you will start to feel better once you exclude gluten. Yes, there may be ups and downs, but the overall trend over the months to come will be of health improvement, possibly starting within days, as your gut mucosa begins to recover and becomes more efficient at absorbing nutrients. Digestive symptoms should ease, as should any tiredness and depression, for instance.

A common concern at this early stage is that you will need a radical overhaul of your diet. Again, a dietitian can explain that this will not need to be the case, that lots of foods are naturally free from gluten, and that the availability of palatable replacement products will mean that your staple meals need not alter drastically – GF pasta can replace wheat pasta; GF breads can replace ordinary loaves.

And, of course, many of these will be available on prescription.

Prescription food

Anyone diagnosed with CD may be entitled to a limited number of staple GF products on prescription, and a dietitian can offer advice in this regard. Your dietitian may stress that it is important to take advantage of any entitlement, as research shows that compliance with the GFD is helped by access to prescription foods, and she may point out that, quite often, prescription products are healthier and lower in fat or sugar than their supermarket 'free from' counterparts.

In Ireland, some tax relief on specialist GF food may be available.

Available products

Products that may be available on prescription include breads, cereals, flour mixes, baking aids, crackers, pizza bases, GF oats and pasta. There are various brands to choose from, with different qualities for different tastes, and the list changes occasionally, with new products added and others removed. The *Food and Drink Guide* itemizes them. Coeliac UK's website has a downloadable list and the society can alert you to updates. The list of products is approved by an independent body, the Advisory Committee on Borderline Substances (ACBS), and it is from this list that your doctor can usually prescribe.

In trying to court new and potentially lifelong consumers, many key suppliers of 'free from' and prescribable foods will send you 'welcome packs' with samples and vouchers – so in some cases you may be able to try before you order.

There are guidelines for the quantities that can be prescribed: in the case of your child this is based on his or her age, and in your case it is based on age, sex, level of activity and, if you're a woman, on whether or not you're pregnant or breastfeeding. The recommendations are given as monthly 'units', with children being entitled to anywhere between 10 and 18 units, and adults between 12 and 18 units. One unit is equivalent to 250 g pasta, 400 g bread, two pizza bases or 200 g crackers, for example.

Take your dietitian's advice when discussing your initial prescription: she may recommend, for instance, products with a higher calcium content if you are calcium-deficient, or foods that can be frozen, or advise against heavy ordering of products with a short shelf-life, all depending on your personal circumstances. Your dietitian can also make a case for you if she feels your allowance should be increased for any reason.

There may, however, be some restrictions, depending on the area of the country in which you live. In England, for instance, only bread and flour mixes are prescribable. The budgets for prescriptions are managed by the local Clinical Commissioning Groups (CCGs) and cutbacks may further impact what your GP may be able to prescribe in your area.

Contact Coeliac UK if you think your prescription has been restricted unfairly, or if you are having difficulty accessing GF foods from your GP.

Getting started

Your doctor will write and sign your prescription, based on the products you have selected within your entitlements, and you can take this to your community pharmacist who will order your food and dispense it to you.

The early months will be in some ways experimental. You can tweak your prescription accordingly, again with the help of your dietitian. Repeat prescriptions are possible, but it's better to wait until you've worked out a selection of foods and a routine that works for you.

There are pharmacy-led local prescription schemes in some parts of the UK, bypassing the need to see a GP. Scotland has a well-established nationwide gluten-free food service, for instance, launched by the Scottish Government.

Cost

Prescriptions are free for children and for some adults, depending for instance on age, income or geographical location. Pregnant women and those with some long-term health conditions do not pay either.

If you do pay, it may be cost-effective to opt for a pre-payment certificate (PPC), available for either 3 or 12 months, which offers unlimited prescriptions. This helps if you pay for other prescriptions as well as your GF entitlements or if you order a variety of product types on prescription.

Controversies and issues

Not all coeliacs obtain food on prescription, and it is a personal decision whether you choose to do so.

Some people don't like the medical connotations of 'illness' that a prescription implies; others don't agree that food should be supplied by the NHS.

The use of Codex wheat starch in certain prescribed foods is criticized by some coeliacs who feel that wheat should be excluded completely from foods labelled 'gluten free'. Others feel that they react to Codex, and indeed some more sensitive coeliacs, especially some children, do appear to have to avoid it.

Those who have to follow a wheat-free or dairy-free diet in addition to a GFD may be unfairly limited in their choices.

Oats in the diet

The situation with regards to GF oats in the coeliac diet is changeable, varies internationally, and is a common source of confusion.

Previous recommendations held that the newly diagnosed should refrain from consuming oats for up to a year, until symptoms had improved and blood tests had normalised, before slowly re-introducing them, and some healthcare providers may still follow these guidelines. Current guidelines from the National Institute for Health and Care Excellence (NICE) state that GF oats can be included or introduced at any point following diagnosis.

Guidelines in the UK no longer specify a maximum recommended intake, but other countries and international bodies sometimes give quantities. 50g a day for adults and a little less for children is generally thought to be safe by those who advocate for oats in the gluten-free diet, and this is the figure typically used when scientists have studied their effects, but a higher intake may well be OK too. The Canadian Celiac Association, for instance, advises up to 70g daily for adults, 25g daily for children, and to 'gradually increase as tolerated'. On the other hand, the Australian and New Zealand coeliac bodies advise that oats should be fully excluded from the GFD until more conclusive research establishes their safety.

The decision is yours, but it's important you receive follow-up monitoring with your dietitian or doctor to ensure any oats you do include are being tolerated. If introducing them, do so very gradually, keep a close eye for symptoms and discuss any issues with your dietitian. Bear in mind that in the first few days after re-introduction or increase, you may experience some change in bowel movements or mild digestive symptoms, which should resolve within a few days. If you increase intake, it is recommended you drink more fluids too, due to the additional fibre in your diet.

Cooking

There is certainly more to coeliac-friendly cookery than merely boiling some rice for your stir-fried vegetables or popping a baked potato into the oven to go with your beans. But before you don your apron and get cooking more adventurously, there are considerations to take care of.

The GF kitchen

If you live alone (or perhaps exclusively with other coeliacs), then you will be able to benefit from 'deglutenizing' your kitchen. Previous baking with ordinary flour might mean there's suspicious white powder lurking in corners, and perhaps breadcrumbs too, so a thorough washing of all kitchen equipment and surfaces is advised.

Toasters can be tough to clean so you will need to replace yours. As for food, give any gluten-containing products to non-coeliacs. Think carefully about where breadcrumbs may be hiding: honeys, marmalades, margarines and other spreads may have crumbs in them if you've 'double dipped' your knife after first applying it to the bread or toast.

The non-GF kitchen

Cross-contamination is a major issue if you are either cooking for non-coeliac family members or sharing with others in a non-GF household.

You will have to be more scrupulous with cleaning, and communicate this importance to the rest of the household. If you can, foster a 'tidying up as you go' approach, rather than allowing unwashed pots and pans, half-eaten bits of food and assorted ingredients to build up, only for gluten to get picked up on fingers and spread further. It will be much easier to keep on top of matters if the kitchen is tidy.

You won't need separate kitchen utensils or other equipment, for the most part. You may need an allocated toaster (although you can use toaster bags), a slicing or chopping board, a bread maker and a bread bin. Reserved cake and biscuit tins are essential. It's wise to have different drainers for different pastas, as they can be tricky to clean properly. You'll also need a no-gluten item of any equipment that isn't washed – such as a wok. Dishes, bowls and cutlery, provided they are washed properly, will be safe.

Should the household give up gluten?

There are advantages and disadvantages to this.

The advantages include easier, quicker and cheaper shopping and less cooking (with no risk of cross-contamination).

The disadvantages are that the GFD is 'imposed' on one or more non-coeliac family members, who may resent it. In the case of children, this could cause problems. Many feel that coeliac children should not be shielded from the realities of a gluten-containing world in this way and that they should learn how to deal with it at home.

A compromise could be best: go GF where you can, make mealtimes mostly GF, encourage non-coeliac family members to take an interest in GF cooking and take care with cross-contamination issues. Most sweet bakery products are equally good in GF forms.

It is ordinary bread and perhaps pasta that non-coeliacs are unlikely to feel they can sacrifice, and these should be accommodated with the usual precautions. Self-contained gluten snacks – such as cereal snack bars – are fine if stored separately and clearly marked for consumption only by non-coeliacs.

That said, some coeliacs do like to have total separation of GF and non-GF, virtually splitting the kitchen into two. Certain products that may be easily mistaken for one another, such as plain biscuits, or that may easily cross-contaminate, such as flours, should be stored separately. Use of prominent labelling or a colour-coding system – perhaps red for non-GF and green for GF – can help here.

It can also help with food: labels on leftovers or for freezer items can avoid confusion. Separate butters and other spreads are recommended. The alternative is a rule where nobody 'double dips' a knife – you included. It may help to go for 'squeezable' options – such as plastic bottles of honey – which can't be contaminated.

Care must be taken when preparing gluten-containing and coeliac-friendly meals at the same time: avoid using the same spoon to stir two different pans of boiling pastas, for example. It's wise to maintain clear separation during cooking. If you have the time, it's better to prepare the coeliac meal first. Regular hand-washing, taking care under nails and jewellery, is paramount throughout.

A lot of the time, once you've taken basic common-sense precautions, you may find that it's best to devise the rules as you go along, learning from trial and error. It may be frustrating at first, but you will get there.

Meals

Avoid thinking of and focusing on the limitations of the GFD – all the foods that you can't cook with and eat. Try to concentrate on what you *can* eat instead – and look upon it as an opportunity to broaden your culinary palate. Having to replace gluten staples with GF varieties and getting to experiment with grains naturally free from gluten can open your eyes to a new world of food. Approach it with a sense of adventure, think creatively, and don't be afraid to make mistakes. You will learn from them. And get better.

Favourite recipes

We all have favourite meals, and there are few recipes that cannot be adapted for coeliacs. For instance, although rice or chickpea spaghetti bolognese or bread and butter pudding made with GF bread may not taste exactly the same as the regular recipes, and your taste buds will take a few weeks to adapt, try not to think of these adapted meals as 'not as good as' they were – just 'different from'. GF versions for most ingredients now exist, so you can find replacements for anything you need.

Great grains

It is important on a GFD to replace the grains you can't eat with the cereals or cereal-like foods you can. You're already likely to be eating rice and may be familiar with polenta or cornmeal, but there are others, and each is nutritious and tasty in different ways.

- Amaranth – a tiny grain, a key crop to the Aztecs. It has a nutty taste, is easily digested and high in proteins, calcium, magnesium and iron, making it ideal for vegetarians and vegans. Cooks in about 15 minutes and should not be overcooked as it quickly turns gooey.

- Buckwheat – despite the name, it is not a wheat and is definitely free from gluten. Popular in Japan, pure buckwheat noodles (soba) make a good alternative to rice noodles and a good substitute for spaghetti. The seeds come in raw form (green) and roasted (reddish-brown). It is commonly used in parts of Russia and China, has a sweet taste, and can be used in casseroles or as a substitute for couscous.
- Millet – a slightly bland cereal of tiny spherical grains, a staple in Africa. It should be cracked by sautéing before cooking, so that it can absorb flavours. Millet flakes can be used as an alternative to oat porridge. It is highly digestible.
- Quinoa – an ancient South American crop, quinoa is a high-protein, complete food, which is nutty, and cooks in around 15 minutes. Use instead of rice or couscous.
- Teff – native to eastern Africa and popular in Ethiopia, this is a tiny, mild and nutty grain, which can be used in soups and stews, as a substitute for bulgur wheat or as an alternative to porridge. It is a nutritious source of iron, calcium, magnesium and zinc.

New recipes

Over time you will want to try totally new meals. You can find inspiration from a number of sources, including cookbooks, magazines, social media and websites (see 'Further reading' and 'Useful addresses').

Baking

You don't have to bake. It can be tough to get right, requiring patience and practice. Gluten imparts elasticity and doughiness and 'bind' to regular bread – making it light, airy and cohesive. Without it, baked products can turn out dense and friable.

GF breads are much tastier than they used to be. Ordinary bakers are branching out into baking for coeliacs, and quality is likely to improve further with increased competition and developments in molecular science. The standard of some smaller speciality producers is exceptional.

If you do want to bake, consider ready-made bread or flour mixes, some of which are available on prescription and just require you to add some staple ingredients.

The bolder will want to be more creative, perhaps invest in a bread maker, and look at experimenting with various flours. A key ingredient in GF baking is a starch called xanthan gum, used to replace the characteristic elasticity of gluten. GF baking powder is widely available.

Getting good results from baking cakes and biscuits is easier – and fun.

Flours naturally free from gluten

Flours each have their own characteristics, and you will come to have favourites. Here are a dozen, with some suggested uses, although most are more versatile:

- arrowroot – good for thickening both savoury and sweet dishes
- buckwheat – for pancakes and crepes, and noodles
- chickpea or gram – for savoury Indian and Asian dishes and flatbreads
- chestnut – for sweet baking (cakes, biscuits)
- cornflour – a thickener, for battering, as meat coating; corn pasta
- mesquite – for sweet recipes or flatbreads
- potato – a savoury thickener (for soups, sauces); for pancakes and waffles
- rice – in all baking and as a thickener; to make rice noodles
- sorghum – for Indian breads and sweet bakery; coating for fried foods
- soy – for egg-free baking; pancake mixes
- tapioca – for sweet and chewy breads and desserts; for thickening sauces
- teff – for savoury breads and sweet cakes.

Eating out

You can't always eat food prepared in your newly safe GF kitchen. There will come a time when you will want or need to consume food prepared by people you don't know at restaurants and other outlets – or indeed order meals for home delivery.

Dining out is one of life's great pleasures, and you shouldn't deny yourself. For many, picking up a quick bite for lunch is a normal part of their working day, and business dinners and family social events are regular events for lots of us.

That said, mistakes are more likely when you're away from home and less in control over the food you eat, so it's not something you can treat lightly or be overconfident about. It is vital to understand what you can and cannot eat – it's unfair to expect others to if you don't.

Where to eat

Ask for recommendations. Fellow, long-standing coeliacs will know of good places, as will your local coeliac group. Coeliac UK has a Venue Guide and offers a GF Catering accreditation scheme to food outlets who meet certain criteria and standards. Many GF bloggers review restaurants and share tips on social media. Most restaurants and chains provide menus online, and many now have dedicated GF menus.

The 'chippie'

With GF batter and careful cross-contamination controls – separate oil and frying areas for fish covered in gluten-containing batter, for instance – many fish and chip shops can now cater for coeliacs, and some hold special events once a week or month where they go entirely GF for the evening or day.

Fast-food chains

Some of the popular fast-food chains' products are listed in the *Food and Drink Guide*, and these chains will gladly give you a list of GF food served.

Pubs

Some pub chains have a GF menu, and some privately owned pubs or 'gastropubs' have good options. It's always worth checking that GF beers are available!

Italian

With pizza and pasta galore, Italian restaurants used to be fairly coeliac-unfriendly in the British Isles, but the situation has improved tremendously in recent years and most high street pizzerias now offer both GF pastas and GF pizza bases. Others may add toppings to your own brought-in GF pizza base – but you must stress that it would need to be baked in a clean oven.

Chinese

Wheat noodles and soy sauce are an obvious source of gluten, but there's also the problem of the tradition of wiping but not washing a wok, causing possible cross-contamination.

Indian

Traditional Indian cooking – especially from the south – is largely GF. Watch out for breads such as naans. Chickpea flour is the usual thickening agent, though, which is naturally free from gluten. Ask about cross-contamination of deep-fried foods. With lots of rice dishes, Indian food can be a good option.

Sushi

A lot of sushi is naturally free from gluten, but do check. Check the crabsticks and soy sauce too.

Sandwich and salad bars

Some sandwich bars have GF sandwiches. In salads, any grain should be checked, but gluten may be 'hiding' in dressings too.

Those bars that allow you to make up your own salads and choose your own dressings are the safest.

Coffee and tea

Cafés and teahouses increasingly stock GF sweet treats and sometimes modest lunch options, and many upmarket hotels now offer GF afternoon tea, with sandwiches and cakes.

Allergen regulations

The particular regulations that apply to non-prepacked foods (see pp. 46–7) apply similarly to food served at outlets such as cafés, restaurants and bars.

Food businesses must provide information on which of the 14 key allergens have been included in the foods they serve, and these must be conveyed in a method appropriate to the business and its clientele. In the case of gluten-containing grains, they will have to provide the name(s) of the cereal(s).

Businesses aren't permitted to make sweeping 'may contain' statements. They should only make one when, following a risk assessment, there is a demonstrable and significant risk of cross-contamination. Neither can they plead ignorance about which allergens are in their products, and the regulations do not oblige food businesses to provide a full list of ingredients (though some may be able to).

There is variation on how the allergens are communicated. Some businesses list allergens 'upfront' – on menus, for instance, or on their counters, with individual notices for each food.

When they choose not to list allergens upfront, businesses must provide clear signposting telling consumers where or how the key information can be found – for instance, by asking a member of staff. This signpost must be provided conspicuously on the menu, on a chalkboard, on a label, or even on a webpage in the case of online ordering.

The option for food businesses to provide the information verbally has caused some concern. The regulations do not stipulate that every member of staff should be able to supply the information, but that there *is* someone on duty who can be called upon to do so. Information provided in such a way must be verifiable in writing – for instance on a chart, matrix or more detailed menu – if you request it.

If you order food from takeaways or other 'distance' sellers via the telephone or internet, allergen information should be made available to you before you place your order, or else you should be informed of how you may obtain it. It must also be made available at the point of delivery, perhaps through labels placed on packaging in which the food is sent.

Gluten free

The same gluten-related claims – such as 'gluten free' – that can be made for prepacked foods and non-prepacked foods can also be made for meals served at food business outlets. The claims can be made on menus, blackboards, webpages or orally, for instance.

Outlets ought to put forward their foods for analytical testing before claims are made, and they should be able to demonstrate that controls remain in place to maintain the low levels of gluten required by law.

Smaller outlets may not be able to afford the testing required on foods and meals to confidently satisfy regulations or meet the requirements of Coeliac UK's accreditation, limiting options for coeliacs. If foods do not contain any gluten-containing ingredients and producers have made every reasonable effort to minimize cross-contamination, they may list such foods or meals under a menu titled 'No gluten-containing ingredients'. If you see such a menu, it is important you make detailed enquiries about how cross-contamination is guarded against, before making a decision to order from it.

Planning ahead

Pre-planning is helpful and reassuring to you; however, more and more chefs and catering staff are now fully aware of CD and understand that it is not a fad diet. You are increasingly likely to find dishes labelled 'gluten free' – if not a dedicated GF menu.

- Phone ahead. Speak with the head waiter or chef, if you can. Try in mid-afternoon during a quiet period. Ask whether those on a GFD can be well catered for, and what may be available.
- Give examples. Explain which kinds of meals are naturally free from gluten or easily adapted to a GFD, such as rice-based

meals and meat, fish and vegetable dishes, and where gluten may 'lurk', such as stock cubes and thickened sauces.

- Satisfy yourself that the kitchen understands cross-contamination issues, e.g. that the spoon used to stir wheaten pasta cannot be used to stir your corn pasta.
- Convey the severity of your condition. Don't just say 'I can't eat gluten', use powerful words: 'I have coeliac disease' or 'Consuming even a trace of gluten will make me extremely ill.'
- Get family, friends and colleagues 'on side' before you go out. Let them know about your dietary needs and that you will need to talk about them, so you don't feel embarrassed when the time comes and they can support you as needed.
- If you're not comfortable with the arrangements and don't feel reassured that you can be safely catered for, then change your plans.

Once you arrive

- If you called ahead, ask to meet the person you spoke with. Go through your conversation again, confirming what you've agreed, reminding the member of staff how serious CD is, about cross-contamination issues, and of the need to check labels on products such as bouillon or condiments that the chef may be using.
- When you arrive at a restaurant which you haven't pre-booked or vetted, inform a member of staff immediately about your requirements. Ask if he or she can check whether there are safe options available. Don't be shy of articulating the precise consequences of errors. Ensure that your conversation is witnessed by members of your party. If you are not confident that the seriousness of your condition is appreciated, don't eat there.
- Read menus carefully. Never let hunger or impatience get the better of judgement. Ask waiting staff to clarify ambiguities and specify safe meals – possibly recommended by the chefs. Some menu items may state 'can be made GF' or similar: ask precisely what changes are made and which precautions are implemented.

- Don't be shy of questioning staff precisely. Is the chef certain of all the ingredients he uses in his recipe? Might a food be cooked in oil previously used to cook an unsafe food? Are separate chopping boards and knives used to prepare different foods? What are the ingredients of the dressings? Have the 'safe' desserts been stored alongside others? Listen carefully to replies.
- Don't become complacent. Go through the usual checks in restaurants at which you've previously dined and that you have come to 'know'. Suppliers, ingredients, chefs, recipes and menus all change. Check every time.
- When your food arrives, use your eyes and nose. Does it look all right? Never pick croutons out of salad, for instance – send it back. Re-confirm with waiting staff that your meal is safe: in busy restaurants, with many clients to attend to, instructions can be forgotten and mistakes made.
- Be polite throughout. Make a point at the end of the meal of thanking staff for catering for you. It will encourage them to become more aware of those with dietary restrictions. Further, spread the word and report excellent establishments to others.

Other catered events and situations

The same regulations that apply to eateries and food businesses selling non-prepacked foods and meals also apply to food served in hospitals, at work canteens, in schools, in prisons, on airlines and at any professionally catered event, such as a wedding or party buffet.

Individuals who provide occasional catering not as a food business – providing food at charity events, for example – are exempt.

Dining at friends'

Being invited to dinner and having to inform your hosts of your condition can feel awkward, but you must impress upon them its seriousness. You may have to explain CD from 'scratch' – what gluten is, where it is found, food labelling, cross-contamination issues, places in which wheat 'lurks' (such as sauces and stock cubes) and so on. It may feel more trouble than it's worth, but good friends will be accommodating and do their utmost to help. Go easy on them: it can be a lot to take in, and some may make mistakes.

Don't be shy of enquiring what your hosts are planning to prepare: 'May I ask what you're thinking of serving? I'm afraid my severe intolerance to gluten restricts what I can eat.'

You could ease your discomfort by offering to help with preparations and cooking, or by bringing your own safe ingredients or prepared dishes that can be microwaved.

5

Food sense: diet and nutrition

It is natural to feel anxious about the impact your diagnosis has had on your nutritional status, and about the continuing effects of your new dietary limitations on your well-being. But it is perfectly possible to eat well on a gluten-free diet – and you may find that you eat more healthily than before.

Eating a healthy diet

So much is written nowadays about eating healthily that you can become overwhelmed with the unnecessarily detailed and sometimes contradictory advice given. It's easy to form the impression that nutrition is complicated. It isn't. In reality, sticking to a few basic principles should ensure that you maintain good dietary habits.

Possibly the most important principle of the GFD is variety: try to eat as diverse a diet as possible. You may not want to spend time fretting over which food offers which nutrient, but you can obtain a wide range by mixing it up as much as possible. Avoid coming to rely on any one 'safe' food that provides only a limited range of nutrients.

How you eat is vital too. Take your time – when you're selecting food, when you're preparing it and most importantly when you're eating it. Eat when you're calm and relaxed and can focus on your meal, not when rushed or distracted, as mistakes are more likely. Remain quietly vigilant and on guard – always. Take care not to become complacent about eating habits – continue to check labelling and to monitor your diet.

Also, don't skip meals, especially breakfast – you'll experience uncomfortable fluctuations in energy levels, and you'll be more vulnerable to casual snacking and grabbing possibly unsafe convenience foods on the go. Plan ahead, and always have good safe foods to hand in case you should be caught short and feel peckish during the day.

Essential foods

Several food groups are key to your daily diet.

Complex carbohydrates

These include all grains, such as rice, quinoa and millet, and the foods based on them, such as gluten-free pastas, breads and cereal products. Potatoes also fall into this category. Roughly eight to ten daily servings for teens and adults and approximately four to seven for children are required to ensure an adequate intake of slow energy-releasing carbohydrates and of fibre. A slice of GF bread, an egg-sized potato, three tablespoons of GF muesli and two heaped tablespoons of cooked rice approximate to a serving each.

Protein foods

Two to three servings of meat, fish, eggs, beans, nuts or seeds are advised. A portion is equivalent to 100 g of meat or fish, two eggs, three tablespoons of beans or a handful of nuts and seeds.

Fruit and vegetables

Fruit and vegetables are essential sources of carbohydrates, fibre, vitamins, minerals and antioxidant chemicals, and you should aim to consume at least five portions daily, preferably more, and in a variety of colours. A handful of berries, an apple, a banana, three tablespoons of peas or lentils and several heaped table-spoons of salad are roughly equivalent to one portion.

Dairy foods

Two or three servings of either milk, yoghurt or cheese are recom-mended by dietitians. A matchbox-sized chunk of hard cheese, a small pot of yoghurt or a glass of milk each provide a serving. Avoid too much cream or butter, as these are high in fat.

Healthy fats

Some fats are needed in the diet, and these may come from some of the foods mentioned above. Unsaturated fats – found in fish (especially oily fish), nuts, seeds, avocados and vegetable oils such as olive oils – are the best.

Water

Two litres daily is the often-quoted figure to which we should supposedly all aspire, but the quantity depends on so many factors – the size of the person, the amount of activity undertaken, the temperature and environment – that it's misleading to generalize.

A good barometer of healthy and adequate hydration is the colour of your urine: too dark signifies that you may lack fluids, so aim to drink enough to keep your pee straw-coloured. Water itself is the best hydrator, but fruit juices, squashes, sodas and milk all contain mostly water and count towards your quota, as do, within reason, teas, coffees and colas. The dehydrating effects of the caffeine in these drinks are hugely exaggerated by some nutritional therapists but research shows they are negligible. Alcoholic drinks, which dehydrate heavily, certainly do not count.

The Eatwell Guide

The Eatwell Guide is a government-backed and evidence-based healthy eating model representing the proportions of food groups that you should aim to consume for a healthy, balanced diet. You can learn more about it at <www.gov.uk/government/publications/the-eatwell-guide>.

The Eatwell Guide principles can be applied to the GF diet, and the approximate percentage shares to aim for are:

- Fruit and vegetables – 40 per cent (at least five portions daily)
- Natural and rendered sources of carbohydrates (potatoes, rice, other GF grains, GF breads and GF pastas) – 38 per cent
- Dairy products / dairy alternatives – 8 per cent
- Protein-rich foods (i.e. meats, fish, eggs and pulses) – 12 per cent
- Oils and spreads – 1 per cent

Supporting messages include to drink 6–8 glasses of fluid daily (water, tea, coffee, sugar-free drinks all count) and to eat high-fat, high-salt and high-sugar foods (such as confectionary, crisps, biscuits and condiments) less often and in small amounts.

Non-essential foods

In moderation, other foods are permitted in the context of a healthy GFD, but take care not to overindulge.

Convenience and snack foods

It's wise to limit your intake of junk foods, desserts, sweet products and processed snack foods, partly because they are high in saturated fats.

Trans fats are a particular class of fats manufactured during hydrogenation – a process that converts liquid vegetable oils into solid fats – and they are often used to prolong shelf-life. They are unhealthier than saturated fats, offer no contribution to nutrition, and are linked to high cholesterol and cardiovascular disease. Typically, trans fats are found in pastries, cakes, biscuits, convenience meat products such as pies and sausage rolls, and some takeaway foods. Be wary of 'free from' foods listing hydrogenated or partially hydrogenated vegetable oil or fats on the label, as well as margarine and 'shortening', as these suggest trans fats. Many manufacturers have a 'no trans fats' policy.

You should also take care with the salt content of nibbles such as crisps (which aren't always GF). Salt can dull the taste buds and contribute to high blood pressure.

Sugary treats

Cakes, biscuits, pastries, chocolate bars, sweets – most of us love occasional treats, and they may be important for your psychological health, especially if you're feeling down about having to exclude gluten. Eat sugar sparingly, though – no more than 5 per cent of your daily calories should come from added sugar, which is roughly equivalent to 30 g – six or seven level teaspoons. Read labels carefully.

Caffeine

Moderate caffeine consumption is safe for most adults, although it can be a mild gut irritant in some. Avoid drinking more than four cups of coffee daily, and remember that black and green teas, cola, cocoa and chocolate products all contain caffeine.

Alcohol

Moderate alcohol consumption – up to two or three units a day, no more than three days a week – is generally considered fine for most adults, and although you may be advised to abstain for a while after your diagnosis while your gut heals on the GFD, there's no reason why you won't ultimately be able to enjoy spirits, wine and GF beers. The health risks of excessive alcohol consumption aside, as a coeliac you need to take extra care as drinking can reduce your vigilance – it's easy to thoughtlessly pop a pretzel from the bar into your mouth when you've had a few more than you should.

'Free from' foods

These have their place, and can be useful, but some products may contain high levels of refined carbohydrates, fats and additives – notably the 'treat' foods. The best products are likely to be prescription staples, some of which are fortified with nutrients.

Coeliac nutrition

Getting you off a gluten-containing diet is the priority when you are diagnosed, but establishing yourself on a nutritionally complete diet comes a close second – joint with the need to resolve any nutritional deficiencies stemming from poor food absorption due to your damaged gut lining that may have been caused by a delay in your diagnosis. These may have been picked up already, but your dietitian may order further blood tests to get a current picture.

Some minerals and vitamins of particular concern are discussed here. Remember that some food recommendations – such as vegan milks, yeast extracts and soya products – will need to be checked for gluten.

Calcium

This is a vital mineral for healthy teeth and bones, and as a result of poor absorption you may be deficient in it and have a need for higher levels in your diet. Your dietitian may also recommend supplements. Long-term low calcium intake can put you at risk of osteoporosis (brittle bones) in later life (see pp. 83–84). Coeliac children do not have an increased need above the ordinary recommended levels.

Foods rich in calcium are:

- all dairy foods
- fortified GF flours and breads
- fortified soya products and tofu
- fortified vegetable milks
- leafy green vegetables
- beans and pulses
- seeds and nuts
- bony fish.

Iron

This is a vital mineral for healthy blood and, again because of poor absorption, you may be iron-deficient and have anaemia. This is of particular concern in teenage girls and young women. Your dietitian is likely to recommend supplements to normalize your iron levels but will also suggest iron-rich foods to incorporate into your diet.

Foods rich in iron include:

- red meat (the richest source)
- oily fish
- egg (especially the yolk)
- fortified GF breads and cereals
- amaranth and quinoa
- dried fruits, such as figs and prunes
- dark green vegetables
- lentils and chickpeas
- soya and tofu
- nuts and seeds.

The absorption of iron can be reduced by tea and coffee, so avoid these with or soon after meals. Absorption can be helped by vitamin C, so it's good to drink juice with an iron-rich meal.

Magnesium

Deficiency in this mineral is common. Magnesium is essential for the formation and maintenance of bones and tooth enamel, and deficiency can increase the risk of brittle bones.

Foods rich in magnesium include:

- fish, meat and dairy products
- amaranth, buckwheat and quinoa
- green vegetables (e.g. spinach, broccoli)
- nuts and seeds
- beans and pulses.

Zinc

This is a 'wonder' mineral in that it has many functions in the body, and many newly diagnosed coeliacs may have compromised levels. It is essential for the digestion of food, for growth and body tissue repair, for immunity and defence, and for sexual health.

Foods in which zinc is found are:

- red meat and poultry
- eggs and dairy products
- shellfish (e.g. oysters, lobster, crab)
- nuts, especially Brazil nuts
- soya and other beans
- wild rice.

B vitamins

The many B vitamins have abundant roles in the body, and there has been concern that coeliac diets are naturally lower in them: substitute products such as GF cereals may not contain as high levels as regular cereals because they are less likely to be fortified with B vitamins.

Folate (folic acid)

Deficiency of this particular B vitamin, common in coeliac disease, may contribute to anaemia, because it is involved in the production of blood cells. Foods in which it can be found include:

- all green vegetables
- corn
- pulses, chickpeas and beans
- oranges
- wild rice and millet.

Vitamin B12

Needed for growth, development and the healthy functioning of the nervous system, vitamin B12 is required in conjunction with folate to produce blood cells, so a deficiency, which is an occasional problem in CD, can also lead to anaemia. Vitamin B12 is found in:

- meats and fish
- eggs and dairy products.

It is not found in naturally vegan foods, so if you don't eat animal products, alternative sources are:

- fortified soya foods and plant milks
- fortified yeast extracts
- fortified margarines.

Vitamin D

Deficiency in vitamin D is another common problem in coeliacs. The vitamin is needed, with calcium, to optimize bone health. It is made in the body by the action of sunlight on the skin, and so a little light exposure daily is important. Good food sources include:

- oily fish
- eggs
- fortified vegan foods (milks, 'cheeses' and margarines).

Vitamin boosts – supplements and injections

Your dietitian will probably recommend that you take some nutritional supplements, at least for a short period. Avoid supplementing without specialist advice, never assume you can compensate for omitted foods with vitamin pills, and don't use supplements as substitutes for skipped meals. Always verify that supplements are GF. Never take additional supplements without letting your dietitian know.

In more serious cases of deficiency, injections of vitamins – for instance, of vitamins B12, D or K – may be recommended.

Weight management

Classical CD patients are often underweight, but these days non-classical forms of CD are more commonly encountered among those newly diagnosed, and many patients are of average weight – or even overweight – at diagnosis.

Once established on a healthy GFD, many coeliacs start to put on weight. This should be generally interpreted as a healthy sign: the gut lining is healing and becoming more efficient at absorbing nutrition and therefore calories. With health improvement comes appetite improvement, further driving caloric uptake.

But if you are overweight, or if you become overweight, you may feel it is a cause for concern, as this can have implications on long-term health and increase your risk of type 2 diabetes and cardiovascular disease.

There is a wide perception that the GFD is automatically healthy, largely as a result of celebrities in the media who speak about having lost weight after giving up gluten. In the everyday world, this is not necessarily the case.

There are obviously steps you can take to control your weight or lose weight if you feel you need to or would like to, and your dietitian can advise. She will probably recommend at least light to moderate exercise: activity is hugely important.

Low glycaemic index foods

The glycaemic index (GI) of a food is a measurement of how it affects your blood sugar levels.

Some foods, those with high GI scores, are digested quickly by the body and so increase blood sugar levels rapidly. In an attempt to 'normalize' these levels, your body releases large quantities of the hormone insulin into the blood. But this can cause a sudden 'dip' in blood sugar, leaving you hungry and lacking in energy. And the result is you eat more.

Instead, many dietitians recommend that you should concentrate on foods with moderate to low GI scores. These tend to be those that your body has to work harder to break down, and that therefore release energy into the blood slowly. These foods are more sustaining and satisfying over a longer period, making it less likely you'll be tempted to eat between meals or make your subsequent meal a larger one than needed, helping with weight control.

High GI foods

These should be consumed in moderation, and include white rice, baked potatoes, sugars, sweets, refined GF cereals, GF treats, white bread and chips or crisps.

Moderate GI foods

These include whole grains (e.g. quinoa, brown rice), GF muesli or oats, GF pasta (better cooked 'al dente'), new potatoes, sweetcorn and a few fruits.

Low GI foods

Examples include brown GF breads, all pulses and lentils, nuts, seeds, dairy produce, most vegetables and many fruits.

Notable from the above list is the high GI value of some of the default GF staples that people typically turn to when diagnosed: white rice and baked potatoes. This is why it's important to incorporate GF grains into your diet.

Fibre

There is some evidence that coeliacs eat less fibre than non-coeliacs and that some GF replacement food is lower in fibre than the regular food. Fibre adds bulk and 'fill' to the diet, helping with weight control. Some tips:

- Choose whole grain GF cereals with, for instance, amaranth and millet.
- Go for brown versions of GF pasta, breads and pizza bases if you can.
- Whole grains such as brown rice, buckwheat and quinoa are important sources of fibre.
- Flours made from gram or chickpea and buckwheat, for example, are more fibre-rich than ordinary GF white flours.

If boosting your fibre intake, remember to keep up your fluid intake.

Sweet treats

Some research indicates that adult female coeliacs have a slightly higher average energy consumption than non-coeliac women, and that this difference is due to sugars in the diet. It is possible that women may be more likely to 'treat' themselves or to overcompensate for the restrictions of a GF diet with more sweet foods. 'Free from' sweet foods may be more calorific.

Obviously, it's a good idea to moderate your intake of sweet and high-fat and calorific treats. A small piece of GF cake or a few GF biscuits a day is probably OK. It's better to restrict them to after a meal, so they don't cause a steep rise in your blood sugar levels. Of course, for occasions, you can enjoy (a little) more.

Probiotics

Billions of bacteria live on the lining of your gut. Weighing in total around a kilogram, these bugs keep your immune and digestive systems working well and help you to digest and absorb vital nutrients, as well as neutralizing any toxins. These so-called 'good' bacteria (or probiotics) also ward off 'bad' bacteria – the pathogens that can cause infection and poisoning.

Research suggests that those on the GFD have slightly poorer populations of gut bacteria, and that coeliacs are more likely to have an overgrowth of non-beneficial bacteria in the gut, which could be responsible for continuing symptoms.

Because modern diets contain few naturally occurring probiotics, there is now a range of food products fortified with them. These include yoghurt products and milk drinks.

The most common probiotics on the market are from the *Bifidobacter* and *Lactobacillus* families, which some experts have suggested offer us better general benefits than other bacterial families and which also seem able to survive the acidic environment of the stomach and the various digestive processes, to reach the large bowel, where they are needed. Studies suggest that they can help to reduce bloating, speed up a sluggish digestive system and support the immune system, but it is becoming increasingly clear that different probiotics have different qualities and can help with different conditions.

There has been some modest research on the possible benefits of probiotics in CD. Research has found that the probiotic *Bifidobacterium lactis* could counteract the toxic elements of wheat gluten and possibly inhibit them from triggering damage to the gut lining. Researchers suggested that probiotics could have value in accelerating gut healing after beginning a GFD, and perhaps even serve as a continuing protective mechanism against coeliacs' almost inevitable low-level gluten intake.

A further study has found that *Bifidobacter* probiotics may offer strong anti-inflammatory benefits to the coeliac gut.

Even though the case for probiotics is far from proven, there is unlikely to be any harm in boosting your diet with them. Supplements are available, but dietary sources include:

- live yoghurts
- fortified yoghurt drinks and fermented milk drinks
- sauerkraut
- miso (check that it is rice or soya miso, not barley miso)
- tempeh.

Weight loss

Weight loss is possible if, as a newly diagnosed coeliac, you find the GFD difficult, unpalatable or depressing. Some people feel wary or suspicious of consuming prescription foods made from Codex wheat starch, or even safe foods, so closely do they relate their diet to their ill health. Understandably, many are frightened of eating out.

Your dietitian will address this with you if she notices a problem, but speak to her if these feelings are familiar. Your dietitian can also help to reassure you of the safety of GF products, increase your confidence and understanding of food labelling so you can choose food confidently, and introduce you to alternative foods, with advice on recipes. A GF cookbook can also inspire you.

Here are some ideas to boost calorie intake in a healthy way via energy-dense, naturally wholesome foods:

- Add seeds and crushed nuts to yoghurts and salads.
- Fortify smoothies with protein powders (e.g. hemp, flax – check they are GF mixes).
- Add rich cheeses, olives and avocado to salads.
- Enrich soups with cream or grated full-fat cheese.
- Stir chopped dried fruits into GF oat porridge.
- Avoid diet or low-calorie products such as diet colas.

Prebiotics

Whereas *pro*biotics are bacteria that promote health, *pre*biotics are indigestible carbohydrates, naturally found in some foods, that feed those friendly bacteria already in your bowel and encourage their proliferation.

A fruit- and vegetable-heavy diet will be richer in prebiotics than a processed- or meat-heavy diet. The known prebiotics are called fructo-oligosaccharides (FOS), inulin and galacto-oligo-saccharides (GOS). They are found generously in chicory and Jerusalem artichokes, and to a lesser degree in garlic, onion, leek, asparagus, GF oats, beans and bananas.

FOS, inulin and GOS are, however, FODMAPs (see p. 116), which some coeliacs may find problematic.

Resistant starch is thought to have prebiotic properties too. This is a type of starch that is not fully digested in the small intestine and that reaches the large intestine, where it becomes available to probiotics. It is present in cold cooked potatoes, green bananas, cold brown rice, beans, pulses, GF oats and yams. Although it is not a FODMAP, some may be sensitive to it.

6
Health issues

In addition to your nutrition, you may also be concerned about other health implications of your diagnosis, of which there may be several.

Other autoimmune diseases

Having an autoimmune disease such as coeliac disease increases the likelihood of having others. Some are quite rare, but a few of the more common ones are considered below. Symptoms should be referred to your doctor.

Dermatitis herpetiformis (DH)

As DH is on the spectrum of gluten-related disorders, a gluten-free diet is the key treatment, but the rash will not clear up quickly with diet alone. A drug called Dapsone can help to get the itchiness of the rash under rapid control, but you may need to take it for up to two years. The side effect of anaemia is fairly common, so this will need to be monitored. Dose reduction can be considered after six months once treatment and the GFD are established.

Type 1 diabetes

This is an autoimmune disease in which the insulin-producing pancreas is damaged. Insulin promotes the body's uptake of sugar from the blood. In its absence, the sugar remains in the blood and does not get used for energy. Symptoms of increased thirst, frequent urination and tiredness result.

Type 1 diabetes is typically diagnosed in childhood, and almost always before CD when they co-occur.

Blood glucose (sugar) control is the cornerstone of treatment, and this will include a diet high in low or moderate GI foods (see p. 75).

One concern for those with diabetes is the level of sugar in some 'free from' products, but it's a myth that people with type 1 diabetes have to give up sugar or sugary foods, although they should be only occasional treats in the context of a healthy diet.

Many people with type 1 diabetes find their glucose levels rising when they move to a GFD, but this is likely to be because their healing gut is absorbing more food. This may mean that you need to adjust insulin replacement quantities.

Thyroid disease

The thyroid is a gland in the neck that produces hormones that regulate metabolism, thermoregulation, nervous system functions, cardiovascular functioning and more. There is a strong link between autoimmune thyroid conditions and CD, and it is worth being aware of possible symptoms and discussing these with your health-care providers should they arise. Stress or pregnancy may be a trigger in some cases.

Graves' disease

This can cause overactivity of the thyroid gland – also known as hyperthyroidism. It is most common among women in their 30s and 40s. Its symptoms are varied and include:

- weight loss
- irritability, feeling emotional
- dislike of heat and warmth
- increased sweating
- swollen thyroid, presenting as a swelling in the neck called a goitre
- bulging eyes or swelling around eyes
- shaking, tremors and rapid heartbeat
- thinning hair.

Hashimoto's disease

This causes chronic thyroid inflammation and underactivity of the thyroid – also known as hypothyroidism. There may be only mild symptoms, if any at all. Others have more notable symptoms, including:

- tiredness
- weight gain
- dislike of cold temperatures
- muscular and joint pain
- slower heart rate
- goitre
- brittle hair and scaly skin
- constipation.

Rheumatoid arthritis

A weak association between rheumatoid arthritis and CD exists. Symptoms are:

- painful or swollen joints
- stiffness in the morning
- weak grip
- tiredness and feverishness.

Sjögren's syndrome

In this relatively common autoimmune condition, the moisture-producing glands in the eyes and mouth are attacked. Other organs may also be affected. Symptoms include:

- dry mouth and sore tongue
- dry and itchy eyes
- vaginal dryness
- digestive problems
- joint and muscular pain.

Crohn's disease and ulcerative colitis

These are serious inflammatory bowel disorders, whose symptoms are similar to those of CD and can be mistaken for a relapse in the condition. Severe diarrhoea or gastrointestinal malaise must always be referred to a gastroenterologist.

Multiple sclerosis

This is caused by autoimmune damage to the nerves of the central nervous system. It produces symptoms such as:

- tingling and numbness
- blurring of vision
- balance and movement problems
- muscular weakness
- tiredness.

Other autoimmune diseases

There are almost 100 autoimmune conditions in total, some extremely rare, with a battery of diverse symptoms, from jaundice and enlarged liver (autoimmune hepatitis) to hazy vision (autoimmune uveitis). There are some symptoms that are common to several of them:

- joint or muscular pain or weakness
- feeling hot or being sensitive to cold or heat
- low fertility and sex drive
- digestive problems
- co-ordination problems and dizziness
- palpitations or an irregular heartbeat
- tingling in the hands and feet
- memory and concentration problems
- depression or mood swings
- dryness of the skin, mouth or hair.

Osteoporosis

One of the most serious and important long-term health considerations in adults diagnosed with CD is osteoporosis – a condition in which the bone mass and density is reduced and bones are more liable to fracture. A huge risk factor is poor absorption of calcium, required for healthy bones, in years of undiagnosed CD.

It is diagnosed via a dual-energy X-ray absorptiometry (DEXA) scan at your local hospital, and this should be advised in those at risk, in order to measure bone mineral density. People at risk include post-menopausal women, men aged over 55 years, the underweight, anyone who has experienced previous fractures, those who have lactose intolerance and those with a family history of the condition. You are more susceptible if you smoke, drink excessively, take little exercise or have a low-calcium diet.

There are a number of recommendations by which you can reduce your risk:

- Stick rigidly to a healthy, calcium-rich GFD.
- Take regular exercise – including weight-bearing exercise.
- Keep to a healthy body weight.
- Keep to within safe alcohol consumption limits.
- Quit smoking.
- Take supplements of calcium or vitamin D, or both – but only if recommended by your doctor or dietitian.

Hyposplenism

This is a reduction in the functioning of the spleen – a small organ on the left side of the abdomen that helps protect against bacterial infections. Hyposplenism is more common in those with CD. Around 30 per cent are affected.

Hyposplenism is usually picked up via blood tests, but people with CD are not routinely assessed for it. Your health practitioner may advise you to be immunized against certain infections to which you may be more vulnerable because of it. The injections may include the flu jab, the pneumococcal vaccine, and the *Haemophilus influenzae* type B (Hib) vaccine.

The charity Coeliac UK now recommends that all coeliacs are vaccinated against pneumococcal infection, with a booster every five years.

Medical treatment

It's likely at some point that you will need to receive medical care unrelated to your CD.

If you, or your child, have to be admitted to hospital for any reason, be aware that your medical team may have very little awareness of CD. Coeliac UK advises you to plan ahead, as some hospitals can find it difficult to cater for those on a GFD. Speak to the charge nurse of your ward or the hospital's dietitian to find out what the hospital can do and whether you need to bring in your own foods. If you don't call ahead, it may take the hospital some time to obtain gluten-free supplies. Be vigilant about any food served to you or your child, and always check it is safe. Anaesthesia has no gluten, and most medicine should be safe too, but always let medics know, just in case. Take some back-up food supplies, and your *Food and Drink Guide*, which may be useful to staff.

By all means let your dentist know you are a coeliac, but there is unlikely to be any product your dentist uses in your mouth that contains gluten.

However, owing to the association between dental enamel defects and CD, especially in children, it is worth letting your child's dentist know about a coeliac diagnosis.

7
Emotional well-being

When there is so much to take on board as a newly diagnosed coeliac – the food-labelling rules, the new food and diet regime, the various physical implications and so on – the psychological impact of your diagnosis may take a back seat. As so much of your time is occupied with the practical implications of your condition, it's easy to neglect your emotional health. So what problems can manifest themselves – and what are the possible solutions?

Coping with diagnosis

Some people welcome their diagnosis. Perhaps after having suffered for years, with doctors unable to get to the root of the problem easily, it can be a relief to be told that the problem isn't all in their heads and is real, and that a gluten-free diet should put them on the road to recovery.

But others don't cope so well. 'Why me?' you may wonder. 'Is it something I did wrong?' Remind yourself that nobody is to blame for coeliac disease: you, or your child, were just unlucky. It was genetics combined with a trigger over which nobody had control.

In an ideal world, as a new coeliac you would react 100 per cent positively, take the diagnosis on the chin, arm yourself effortlessly with a wealth of knowledge on the condition, and experience no emotional hiccups in making the transition to a gluten-free lifestyle.

But this is real life, and most people, through no fault of their own, find the road to acceptance a bumpy one, much like a bereavement.

Shock, anger, disbelief

You may feel fury that your body has let you down, perhaps that you're still young, that it shouldn't be 'failing' you already. You may find the diagnosis difficult to believe and the implications too huge to contemplate: 'It cannot be true!' Perhaps you feel anger at the situation in which you find yourself, anger at how much you're going to miss out socially and food-wise, anger at the glutenous society, filled as it is with newly banned foods such as pizzas and cakes, which have suddenly become unavailable to you. You may take your frustration out on loved ones.

Letting your feelings show can be beneficial in the short term. It is normal and it will usually pass quickly, and those close to you will, it is to be hoped, understand.

Denial and indifference

'I don't have to worry about reading labels or watching what I eat – my mother will make sure I eat the right things.'

'I know I've got to cut down on gluten – but I can still have a few biscuits with my tea in the afternoon.'

'I've managed fine up till now. I can put up with the diarrhoea, take some Imodium, and will just carry on as before. It can't be that serious.'

Do you recognize any of the above attitudes?

Passing the buck for your care on to others, not taking the diagnosis seriously, adopting a reckless attitude towards your well-being – these are all possible initial responses that need to be tackled, especially if they linger.

Self-pity

A brief period spent feeling sorry for yourself can do you good: if you're overwhelmed with your diagnosis and its implications, having a short 'shut down' for a few days could be just what you need and is perfectly normal. Allow yourself time off work. When you emerge from the gloom, as you begin to accept your situation, you will probably find yourself ready to face the task head on.

Continuing problems

Some people take CD in their stride. Others experience occasional or chronic psychological difficulties, and it is vital to be aware of these.

Depression

This is a symptom of undiagnosed CD, but one study found that diagnosed coeliacs on a GFD were more likely than the general population to be depressed. A short period of mild depressive withdrawal can act protectively. But when this stretches on indefinitely, the situation becomes serious.

Older people, a group in which diagnosis rates are rising sharply, may be particularly susceptible to the 'coeliac blues'. You may be feeling doubly fragile at a time when your body might already be showing other signs of 'wear and tear'. This vulnerability can be much more debilitating than the practical implications of suddenly having to avoid wheat. Feeling 'set in your ways' and unable to make adjustments may also bring you down.

Symptoms of depression include:

- indifference, including to pleasurable activities
- reduced appetite or reduced interest in food
- lethargy and tiredness
- disordered sleep patterns
- poor concentration and motivation
- feelings of inadequacy or hopelessness
- loss of self-confidence.

Complacency

This is a sign that denial could be creeping back. Ask yourself these questions:

- Have you taken to being cavalier with checking food labels?
- Are you beginning to take risks with products carrying 'may contain' warnings?
- Have you started to catch yourself wondering, 'I've been healthy for ages – how much can it hurt, just this once?'
- Do you increasingly avoid telling people about your condition when you should do so?
- Have you skipped appointments with your doctor or dietitian?

A 'glutening' episode can act as the wake-up call in this situation, but it is preferable to identify any slide towards complacency and nip it in the bud.

Lingering denial

'I've been gluten-free for three months, so I deserve that piece of cake.'

'I wasn't very ill. My body will have recovered now and I'm young and healthy so it doesn't matter if I stray every now and then.'

The problem with continuing denial about the realities of CD is that it can, clearly, lead to straying from the diet and exposing your gut to gluten. Naturally, it's tempting. You may desperately miss 'real' bread. You may get offered a piece of birthday cake in the office and want to enjoy it with everyone else. It's very, very hard.

Embarrassment

Sadly, many coeliacs feel ashamed of their condition, and embarrassed at feeling as if they're 'making a fuss' at social events. People are not always understanding or sympathetic: because the GFD is adopted misguidedly by some people as a means through which to lose weight or 'detox', you may be treated sceptically as a dieter or faddy eater.

Coeliacs can react to this in one of two ways: either they avoid social situations and isolate themselves, or they expose themselves to risks by not speaking up.

Anxiety and stress

Even if you were relieved at your diagnosis, that relief may be short-lived: the stress of not knowing what was wrong and perhaps trying to convince your doctor that something was amiss may have been lifted, but now it has been replaced with the anxiety of an uncertain future. How are you going to cope? *Can* you cope?

Some underlying anxiety is OK: you need to be alert to possible danger and ready to respond. For instance, it is vital that you maintain a low, constant level of vigilance to avoid gluten, so don't look upon stress as all bad.

That said, chronic stress can be debilitating: it is often felt in the gut – the last place you want disturbance as a coeliac – and is a sign of a problem that needs to be addressed.

Symptoms of anxiety include:

- a dry mouth
- cold or hot sweats
- changes in eating habits
- inability to work or concentrate
- sleep disturbance
- low libido or sexual dysfunction
- obviously untrue negative thoughts.

Schizophrenia

Schizophrenia is a mental health illness, affecting thinking, feeling and behaviour. Age of onset is typically in the teenage or young adult years. Schizophrenia may involve disordered thoughts, delusions, hallucinations, apathy and lack of emotional response and interest.

A link between CD and schizophrenia is controversial but has been the subject of speculation since the 1960s, when a researcher made the observation that it was rare in communities that consumed no wheat. The link is suspected by some, but if it exists the true nature of it remains unclear, although autoimmune mechanisms may be involved.

Studies have found around a third of those with schizophrenia have high levels of antibodies to gluten in their blood, and the basis for gluten as a trigger to some cases of schizophrenia is being explored.

Some people with schizophrenia may benefit from a GFD.

Eating disorders

A possible association between CD and eating disorders such as anorexia nervosa and bulimia nervosa has received very little attention.

The causes of eating disorders are difficult to pinpoint, but biological, environmental and psychological factors are all likely to be involved. They are more common in younger women, but are not exclusively seen in this group.

You are more susceptible if you are anxious or depressed or have low self-esteem, or have experienced a stressful event. Some researchers think the Westernized ideal of thinness and the obsession with weight loss and celebrities or models can be a contributing factor. It would not be implausible that the weight gain in response to a GFD that many coeliacs experience could be a potential triggering issue for some women – and indeed young men.

It is also possible that the great care that coeliacs need to take with their diets may, in vulnerable people, gradually slip towards hyper-obsessiveness, increasingly restricted diets and then anorexic behaviour.

Becoming obsessed with diet or size, being disturbed by minor weight gain, depression, social withdrawal and excessive exercise are all signs of a problem.

Self-help

So what can you do? Although there are plenty of ordinary people, specialists and groups who can help, there's one person who is undoubtedly the most important in your own emotional care and personal journey towards acceptance of your CD. You.

Positive learning

Learn everything you can about CD and approach your fact-finding mission positively; your aim is to eliminate the anxiety that ignorance breeds.

If there is something that you do not understand about CD, a niggling query that is bothering you, then resolve to find the answer – if this book can't help, ask a health-care professional or contact Coeliac UK. Getting on top of issues about which you're unsure is empowering.

Positive thinking

Remind yourself that your condition, despite being serious, is manageable. Focus on the positives: think of the foods that you can eat (there are hundreds), not those that you can't (there are only a handful); think of how your health will improve, not worsen, on a GFD.

Positive thinking also helps your self-esteem and self-confidence, vital when facing the gluten-containing world as a coeliac.

Exercise and activity

Good for you physically but super on a mental level too. You don't have to join a gym. Don't run if you hate running. Merely resolving to take more walks is effective. Instead of focusing on the 'exercise' aspect, do something you love that involves activity and energy – such as amateur dramatics or DIY. Your body was designed to be active through living.

Fun and laughter

Humour is subjective, and what makes you laugh may make someone else scratch their head, but take part in fun activities, watch your favourite comedy shows to cheer yourself up and share a joke with fellow coeliacs – whether it's over a dodgy coeliac tummy or the silly things that 'wheaties' (non-coeliacs) say.

Laughter is not the best medicine – nutritious GF food is – but it's still a very good one!

Pride

Why not? What's the alternative – shame?

Most people avoid certain foods. This can be for any number of reasons – ethical positions, religious beliefs, cultural sensibilities, food allergies, food intolerances, unpalatability, health concerns. You don't eat gluten for a very good reason – and it's as valid as others' reasons for not eating peanuts, dairy or pork, for example. Have the same pride and confidence in your restriction as anyone else.

And if you don't want to always wear your 'coeliac hat'? That's OK too. You can be discreet – as long as it doesn't compromise your health.

Relaxation and breathing

Many people say they're unable to relax, but there is more to unwinding than just willing yourself to do so. Pampering – a hot bath, aromatherapy oils – can help, as can a massage from a willing partner. Meditation, prayer and chanting are deeply relaxing if they are right for you personally, as are forms of yoga and healing martial arts such as t'ai chi. Find what works for you, and remember that relaxation takes practice.

For instant stress relief if you're feeling tense or nervous, try a technique of 'expanding' your peripheral vision. Find a point opposite you, just above eye-level, and keeping your eyes on that point, begin slowly to broaden your field of vision to notice more of what's on either side of the point, so that eventually you're paying attention to what is visible in the corners of your eyes. You should begin to feel your breathing moving lower in your chest, slowing down and becoming deeper, and your facial muscles relaxing. Very calming.

Indeed, learning to breathe correctly is of enormous value to stress relief: inhale deeply and slowly into the belly to the count of three, exhale evenly to the count of three, then pause for one – and repeat. Yogic breathing while seated and focusing on a lit candle is soothing.

Volunteering

Helping yourself by helping others can work wonders. Volunteering gives something back to the community, and will also strengthen your character and prove fulfilling.

Coeliac UK is always looking for volunteers to help with campaigning and research or to boost local support group membership and activities. The charity also supports members in organizing fundraising events. You could also get involved in educational activities: giving a demonstration of GF baking at your local school to kids, parents and teachers, for instance.

Volunteering can put you in touch with other coeliacs who can offer moral and practical support too.

Another option might be to volunteer to be a media 'case study': medical journalists often require these to illustrate articles in lifestyle magazines and newspaper health sections. CD is a popular subject, partly because it is so underdiagnosed, and there is a constant need for new case studies. They offer a chance to share your story: this can be therapeutic and may perhaps help readers to solve their own health predicaments. All that is usually required is a short telephone conversation with a journalist, and possibly a photograph.

Writing

Putting your anxieties and fears down on paper is an excellent way of clearing your head, unburdening yourself, understanding your problems and charting your emotional progress.

An alternative to keeping a private diary is keeping a public one – or a 'blog', which can be an online web diary of your experiences with CD and, well, anything you like. Coeliac blogs are very popular, and many coeliacs share their tips, recipes, product reviews and thoughts online and invite you to add comments. You may find your blog attracting attention from coeliacs worldwide. Comment on others' blogs and they're more likely to comment on yours.

Friends and family

The role of loved ones in your emotional care should never be underestimated. When you're first diagnosed, assess your support network and 'rally the troops' – your core group of partner, friends and family, who care for you and who you know can help you to come to terms with your condition.

The good guys

You need around you positive people who can offer practical advice and emotional support, who can lift your gloom and bring laughter into your life when you feel there is none, and who make you feel understood. The most valuable are the people who know your needs and the implications of your illness, who don't make you feel like a burden, who can act as your personal 'bodyguards' should you be tempted to stray from the diet – and who don't make demands in return.

You also need people who are unafraid to give you difficult truths when they apply – to point out that you are foolishly taking risks with certain foods, or that you may benefit from seeking professional help with your mental health, for instance.

Shutting people out is a never-win situation. Most who care for you will want to help in any way they can, so don't be too proud to ask for practical help or a shoulder to cry on. You may feel you want to protect family members from the difficulties and implications of your CD, but, again, most prefer to be involved – even if it's just by helping you out with the GF groceries.

The not-so-good guys

Understand that not everyone you meet, work with or are friendly with will be helpful or supportive, often through ignorance, not malice. Some people simply will not 'get' CD, refusing to believe that something as innocuous as wheat can make you so ill, and will insist that 'allergies are all in the mind' because an article they once read said so. Upsetting as this may be, it will probably always be the way to some extent, and arguing the case may not always prove fruitful or make you feel better.

All friends have strengths and weaknesses, and much-valued confidantes may not necessarily be the right ones to turn to when you're suffering problems related to your CD; for instance:

- those who enjoy the 'fuss' of your CD, making an exaggerated issue of it at restaurants, for example;
- those who trivialize your condition and say you shouldn't take it so seriously; or
- those who 'hijack' your CD with their health problems less serious than your own.

Be aware of different people's reactions and be alert to those who make you feel worse. There's no shame in taking a step back if you need to. You must come first.

That said, remember too that people are more likely to be understanding and supportive if you demonstrate that you take your CD seriously. If you're a little reckless with label-reading or if you 'cheat' occasionally for a special occasion, people are understandably more likely to be sceptical.

Support groups

Occasionally, you may feel more comfortable seeking the support of strangers.

Charities

The Coeliac UK helpline (0333 332 2033) is staffed by knowledgeable people who can offer emotional as well as practical support. Other support lines of potential value include:

- Samaritans – 116 123
- Anxiety UK Helpline – 03444 775 774
- Beat (eating disorders association) – 0808 801 0677.

Even if you don't volunteer, taking part in local activities organized through Coeliac UK's support networks will relieve the isolation you may be feeling as a newly diagnosed coeliac.

Online support

Online forums dedicated to those with CD – or other food-related sensitivities – can be supportive. People who live in remote areas, those who are disabled and single parents of young children are among those who find these groups of particular value – but they can help anyone who perhaps is shy or has difficulty with face-to-face contact, and prefers the anonymity the internet offers.

Although groups can be encouraging, choose one with a knowledgeable moderator, who will remove suspect, offensive or dangerous postings. It is better to use them for matters such as emotional support, advice on food products, sharing recipes and tips on where to eat – but not medical advice.

There are wide supportive networks and communities on social media platforms such as Facebook and Twitter too. 'Like' or 'follow' coeliac groups, GF bloggers, 'free from' commentators and specialist dietitians, and they will often return the compliment – especially if you engage meaningfully with them. Many are very generous with their advice and knowledge, and genuine friendships are regularly struck up through social media. Many coeliacs turn first to the internet when they need someone to offer emotional support.

The bonus in making use of the internet is that it can keep you up to date with developments in the world of CD and GF – medical research, newly published articles, new food launches, and so on.

Professional help

Sometimes, stubborn psychological problems need to be referred a step further.

Your GP

Doctors are your first port of call if you're suffering symptoms of stress, depression or anxiety or are concerned with other areas of your psychological health. Doctors are trained to see signs of emotional difficulties in their patients and ideally placed to advise on possible private treatments or referrals. Do make use of your GP; many have good counselling skills and unburdening yourself to your GP may be all you need.

Your dietitian

If you're anxious about gluten avoidance or about nutrition, your dietitian can help fill the gaps in your knowledge and offer guidance and reassurance. Dietitians may also have a role to play in identifying and helping resolve possible eating disorders. Tempted to eat a gluten-filled treat? Missing bread? They can support and advise here too.

Your gastroenterologist

Your most complex queries can almost certainly be answered by your gastroenterologist. The more knowledge you demonstrate and the more questions you ask of specialists, the more likely you will be given greater detail and reassurance.

If you feel burdened by not knowing whether or not you are improving on a GFD, a consultant can arrange a biopsy to check for gut recovery. If you feel tempted to stray from the diet, a gastroenterologist can remind you of the seriousness of the damage you risk – that there's only so much recovery your gut can take, and that you're increasing your long-term risks of complications such as osteoporosis and malignancies.

Life coaches

Increasingly popular, a life coach can help with motivation to change your lifestyle to benefit your health, give you confidence to talk to people about your dietary needs, and set goals towards making important changes fast and less urgent ones gradually over time.

'Talking' therapists

If your doctor feels that you need more specialized help, referral for counselling or psychotherapy may be suggested. There are not many specialists working in these fields in the NHS, so a private referral may be required.

There are few differences between the talking therapies, even though counselling sounds – and is – gentler and less demanding than psychotherapy. Both involve face-to-face meetings with a trained therapist to reach any number of end goals, depending entirely on the patient, such as the reduction of psychological distress and the promotion of emotional health.

Counsellors will listen to you, aim to identify with you and your dilemmas, help you to clarify them in your mind, and perhaps give advice – although generally their aim is to guide you to discover your own answers to your problems through carefully guided discussion. Counsellors can, for instance, help patients to cope and come to terms with difficult events like diagnosis.

Psychotherapists, of which there are many kinds, work similarly, but use more analytical approaches and explore difficulties in greater depth. They may work with those suffering from depression, anxiety and addictive behaviour disorders, those who are finding it difficult to adjust to their illness and those whose condition is having an impact on many areas of their life.

Make sure you have an assessment session, and discontinue any therapy with a specialist with whom you feel uncomfortable – being at ease with your counsellor is vital. Remember too that counselling is not easy or a magic wand: expect positive changes but not miracles. Some people approach therapy expecting their stresses to be entirely removed, but therapists will not do this: they will arm you with coping mechanisms, not seek to abolish all your responses.

The road to acceptance

Resolve to take positive action – learn to scrutinize labels, ask questions, learn everything you can about CD.

Focus on everything positive – there are lots of new foods to enjoy, remember how much healthier you feel on the GFD, remind yourself you are on the road to recovery.

Forgive yourself – if you make mistakes, if you feel grumpy, if you need some time to yourself.

You are never alone – spend fun time with loved ones, talk to fellow coeliacs, call a support charity if you need one.

Cognitive behaviour therapy (CBT)

CBT is an objective psychotherapeutic approach that is less interested in what caused your emotional or psychological difficulties and more concerned with how you handle your dilemmas. It challenges negative thought patterns, helps you to identify and understand them, equips you with coping skills and implements changes to unhelpful thinking or behaviour. The therapy is structured, practical and result-focused, unlike counselling, which usually involves 'freer' conversation and a greater rapport with the therapist.

CBT might be right for those looking for help with a specific issue. It is useful for depression, phobias or stress, for example, where the emphasis may be on cognition or thinking, while for eating disorders, predominantly behavioural issues will be tackled.

Hypnotherapy

This is a psychotherapy that uses hypnosis – a state of deep relaxation and heightened awareness, which makes the mind more receptive to positive suggestion. It can help those suffering from low self-esteem and anxiety, to name but two.

8
Practical issues

Coeliac disease may have an impact on other areas of your life as well.

Holidays and travel

You may feel nervous about travel, especially overseas, but by taking sensible measures there's no reason why you can't enjoy a trip anywhere, whether for business or pleasure.

Coeliac UK offers a number of resources, including leaflets on travelling to several dozen countries, with some useful phrases in translation. The charity carries advertising for many travel companies and hotels in its *Live Well Gluten Free* magazine, and it can also recommend an insurance policy.

If travelling to Europe, apply for a European Health Insurance Card – see <www.ehic.org.uk> – before you travel. It entitles you to medical treatment should you need it, but is not a replacement for travel insurance.

Research

Find out about your destination's food culture before you travel – some nations use little wheat (countries in the Far East), whereas others use it abundantly (most European nations).

If you're undecided where to go, bear in mind that although it may seem more logical to travel to a place where gluten grains are rarely used in the cuisine, in reality people in countries in which wheat or rye are common may be more likely to be coeliac-aware. Scandinavian nations, Ireland and Italy are good examples.

Holidaying in the UK or Ireland has obvious advantages. Many hotels are now promoting themselves as 'coeliac friendly' (or 'allergy friendly') and actively encourage those with food sensitivities to stay.

Self-catering accommodation is an option, but if you're travelling somewhere rural check that you have easy access to a supermarket or store offering basic essentials.

Booking

If organizing your travel through an operator, let them know about your requirements – they may be able to make recommendations and will certainly try to accommodate you as much as possible.

When booking flights, specify that you need a gluten-free meal. Ask whether you can take GF food supplies in your luggage – a request that you may need to support with a medical note from your doctor. You may be able to increase your baggage allowance if you explain to the airline in advance. Consider packing toaster bags too.

Some countries have strict quarantine policies. For instance, Australia and New Zealand will allow you to bring certain GF staples in your luggage, but you must declare them and be prepared for them to be inspected on arrival.

Travelling

Have some snacks with you for whatever journey you undertake: finding GF options at motorway services, stations and airports is not always easy. Good options include homemade sandwiches made with GF bread, GF crackers, GF cereal bars, rice cakes, dried fruit and bananas.

Introduce yourself to cabin crew and remind them you requested a GF meal or snack when you booked.

Food labelling

The rest of the EU is subject to the same labelling legislation as the UK and Ireland. Here are some terms to look out for on food products:

- English: 'gluten-free' or 'very low gluten'
- German: *'glutenfrei'* or *'sehr geringer glutengehalt'*
- Dutch: *'glutenvrij'* or *'met zeer laag glutengehalte'*
- French: *'sans gluten'* or *'très faible teneur en gluten'*

- Italian: *'senza glutine'* or *'con contenuto di glutine molto basso'*
- Spanish: *'sin gluten'* or *'muy bajo en gluten'*
- Portuguese: *'isento de glúten'* / *'sem glúten'* or *'teor muito baixo de glúten'*.

In the USA, as well as 'gluten free', expressions such as 'without gluten' and 'free of gluten' are also permitted. They refer to products with no more than 20 parts per million (ppm) of gluten.

Australia and New Zealand are unusual. Foods labelled 'gluten free' must contain 'no detectable gluten' (about 3 ppm according to the best detection tests) – considerably less than allowed elsewhere. However, you may see a Crossed Grain symbol on products, not labelled gluten free, which do meet international Codex standards of 20 ppm. The situation here is changeable, and their stricter labelling rules may be slightly relaxed in future as detection tests continue to improve.

Outside those nations – in Africa and Asia, for instance – labelling may be less specific and more unreliable. However, you may occasionally be pleasantly surprised. Food labelling law in Brazil, for instance, specifies that the gluten status must be declared on all food and drink.

Remember that a particular brand or product that is safe in your home country might *not* be so in another nation.

Eating out

In most countries where English isn't spoken you should still be able to find an English menu. Dietary cards explaining your requirements are available from some organizations if there is a language barrier issue, and may be worth ordering in advance. Often the best source of recommended coeliac-friendly eateries is the country's coeliac charity (see 'Useful addresses').

Working life

Your CD should not hamper your working life or career choice – unless, perhaps, you wish to be a beer taster or restaurant reviewer! There are, for instance, plenty of successful athletes who are coeliacs.

Some jobs in which you may eat 'on the job' – pilot or flight attendant, for example – may require special provisions for your food, but as these are increasingly provided for passengers, again there shouldn't be a special problem.

Tell your employer that you have CD. If you need to take time off for health appointments or if you've been 'glutened' and need to take a few days off work, your employer is likely to be more understanding if already aware of your condition.

The armed forces

The one exception is the armed forces. Those with CD are not recruited because a guarantee to provide for a gluten-free diet in the field or on operations is not feasible, says the Ministry of Defence. Those diagnosed while serving will, where possible, be offered an alternative role or, if not, a medical discharge.

Beauty and grooming

Every day we wash, scrub, cleanse, moisturize, deodorize and condition parts of our body with a selection of gels, soaps, sprays, creams, colours and powders. Some of them may well use gluten-containing grains. How safe are they?

This is difficult to answer as little research has been conducted. You will often hear quoted that a large proportion – up to 80 per cent – of what we apply to our skin is absorbed into the body. This is exaggerated, and it varies depending on the product and the individual.

Lipsticks and lip balms are perhaps a more valid concern as they come into contact with the mouth, and trace amounts may be absorbed more readily and swallowed. Occasionally these products can contain ingredients derived from the gluten grains. All the major commercial brands of toothpastes and mouth washes avoid gluten-containing ingredients, and the same goes for most 'natural' brands of toothpaste, whose packaging may confirm this.

While the risk in the cases of lip products is unclear but likely to be small, it is understandable that some coeliacs feel that they want to exclude gluten grains totally from their life regardless, and so may choose to adopt a no-gluten policy when it comes to their toiletries.

Product labelling

Although only foodstuffs, and not cosmetic items, are bound by food allergen directives and there are no specific rules for labelling gluten, ingredients must by law be listed on personal care products – either on the container or on the packaging. Cosmetics that are small and difficult to label clearly are partially exempt; instead, their ingredients should be displayed close to the item's point of sale or be available on a leaflet.

That said, botanicals sometimes appear solely in Latin, without English translations. Here are the ones that matter:

- Barley – *Hordeum* or *Hordeum vulgare*
- Oat – *Avena sativa*
- Rye – *Secale cereale*
- Wheat – *Triticum* or *Triticum vulgare*.

Grains tend to crop up in products of a thicker consistency, such as lip products, gels, creams and exfoliating scrubs, but occasionally deodorants too. Wheat proteins are common in haircare products, as they are excellent at conditioning.

Reactions to cosmetics

Reactions to cosmetics are common and it is easy to assume that gluten may be a culprit, but it is unlikely.

Contact dermatitis, characterized by red itchy patches of skin, is the most common reaction. It is usually non-allergic and triggered by an irritant such as an abrasive or a detergent. The reaction is delayed, not immediate, localized to the site of application, and usually caused by repeated exposure to the cosmetic rather than one-off use. Those with eczema and very light-skinned people are more susceptible.

Allergic contact dermatitis is less common. It is often caused by one or more of the many thousand fragrances found in bodycare products, but also by preservatives, ultraviolet filters and emulsifiers. Unlike irritant contact dermatitis, allergic contact dermatitis can spread beyond the site of application.

Immediate 'nettle' rashes are occasionally reported too, and it is known that these can be caused by hydrolysed wheat protein, among many other substances.

If you experience what you think may be a reaction to cosmetic ingredients, it is worth seeking your GP's advice and a possible referral. Patch testing by a dermatologist can help identify culprits in contact dermatitis, and allergy testing may be appropriate for other suspected reactions. Don't self-diagnose, as it is easy to be mistaken and you may leave yourself exposed to ingredients that you continue to react to.

Other non-food exposures

Communion wafers

If you're a Roman Catholic or Anglican, you may be concerned about Holy Communion. Roman Catholic doctrine specifies that the eucharistic wafers must be unleavened, made from wheat and contain a trace of gluten. The Church of England position is similar, though leavened bread is permitted. Despite some reports that these churches 'ban' GF hosts, wafers made with Codex wheat starch, which fulfil the key criterion, and contain very low levels of gluten, are perfectly valid eucharistic matter at both. It is 'naturally' GF hosts, made with rice and potato, for example, which are not considered bread.

Other Christian churches, such as Mormon, Methodist or Baptist, typically aren't as strict, and may allow wheat-free and GF wafers and even ordinary commercial or homemade breads to be used.

Coeliac UK's website lists Communion wafer suppliers in the UK, and suppliers are also noted in the Coeliac Society of Ireland's *Food List*. Speak to your church in the first instance, as they may have supplies already in stock or be able to help order on your behalf.

If GF hosts prove too difficult, consecrated wine counts as Communion, although not all churches offer it routinely. Bear in mind that cross-contamination may be an issue too – if, for instance, a piece of 'ordinary' host is dipped into the chalice as part of the consecration. Speak to celebrants about possible solutions.

Pet food

Most dog and some cat food contains wheat as a filler. It's unlikely this will find its way into your mouth, but it is worth washing your hands carefully after handling and cleaning up carefully after your pet has been feeding.

Stationery

Envelope gum and any gum on lickable stamps is free from gluten.

9
Children and family

It is impossible for home life not to be impacted by coeliac disease when at least one member of the family has the condition. First-degree relatives of those with CD are ten times more likely to have it themselves, so it is natural to be concerned about all loved ones – especially children.

Pregnancy and birth

There is an increased risk of fertility difficulties as an undiagnosed coeliac, so if you are trying to conceive, are pregnant for the first time or are pregnant again following a miscarriage, you may be naturally nervous about carrying a child to term. Rest assured that a strict gluten-free diet should soon normalize your fertility levels and that there are no increased risks to you or your unborn child as a coeliac mum-to-be who adheres to the diet.

Before conceiving

If you're planning a pregnancy, discuss it with your health-care advisers. It may not be advisable to try to conceive soon after your diagnosis if you have a compromised nutritional status.

Your intake and levels of folic acid (folate) are key. You may be deficient in this B vitamin, and all women are advised to supplement with 400 micrograms of folic acid daily as soon as they stop using contraception and to increase their intake of folic acid with, for example, green vegetables. Women with CD may need a little more, so speak to your dietitian. Folic acid helps to prevent neural-tube disorders such as spina bifida in your unborn child.

During pregnancy

General healthy eating guidelines, many outlined in Chapter 5, apply to all mothers-to-be too: at least five portions of fruit and vegetables daily, lots of gluten-free starches and grains, plenty of fluids, moderate caffeine intake – but no alcohol.

Calcium intake is particularly important in pregnancy, especially in coeliac mums, and low-fat dairy products are recommended.

Similarly, iron intake, too, is key – meats, fish, eggs and pulses supply iron, as well as vital protein. Only supplement with iron on medical advice. Try GF crackers or rice cakes if you need to nibble something to help with morning sickness.

The Department of Health advises all women to avoid certain foods in pregnancy:

- raw and partially cooked eggs
- raw shellfish and meats
- blue-veined and soft-ripened cheeses
- pâtés
- shark, marlin and swordfish
- liver and liver products.

Your prescription entitlement increases modestly in the third trimester of your pregnancy, so take advantage of this and review the foods you need with your dietitian.

Childbirth

There are no particular considerations for coeliac women in childbirth, although some studies suggest that giving birth naturally rather than via Caesarean section slightly decreases the likelihood of your child developing CD in later life.

Early feeding

Exclusive breastfeeding in the first six months is recommended, although studies suggest very few women follow these guidelines. There was some research suggesting that breastfeeding could offer some protection against the development of CD later on in high-risk babies, but later studies have suggested this may not be the case.

You are entitled to additional units of prescription food when breastfeeding. Formula milk provides all the nutrition your baby needs, and all is GF.

Weaning

Some babies aren't satisfied with a milk-only diet until six months and may need to start solids a little sooner – but never before four months. Discuss this with your midwife or health-care adviser.

Gluten should not be introduced into any baby's diet before six months. Delaying it beyond this period does not seem to reduce the eventual risk for developing CD, but it may delay its onset.

Coeliac UK advises that once a baby is established on solids, gluten should be given regularly, since CD can only be diagnosed once it is a routine part of the diet. Should symptoms occur (see p. 3), they are usually obvious at this young age.

The weaning and breastfeeding advice to babies at higher risk of CD is subject to change owing to continuing studies in this area, so always take definitive up-to-date advice from Coeliac UK or your health-care advisers.

Children and CD

If you have a child who is newly diagnosed with CD you may feel a mix of emotions: protective, anxious, fearful, relieved. It may be some consolation to know that children are tough little things who adapt superbly to the new requirements – possibly because they won't consider their diet to be a priority in their lives at that age. At a time when they're still growing and developing, lasting damage caused by poor absorption of food and malnutrition is very unlikely.

It's generally good advice to focus on the present – do what you need to do *now* – and cross certain bridges when you come to them.

If your child is diagnosed with CD you will have access to a specialist paediatric dietitian who will be best placed to advise on any nutritional concerns. There are no specific recommendations for coeliac children, but she will ensure that you understand the need for a healthy GFD and an adequate intake of such minerals as calcium and iron. Some children may have anaemia on diagnosis, so this will be addressed.

If diagnosed in infancy, your child may not have been exposed to too many gluten-containing foods, and so he or she may not be too concerned with (or even notice) the sudden change in diet. Your child may, though, have made the connection with having felt sick and the previous diet. You will need to talk to your child at some point – the sooner the better – and this really depends on the level of maturity and when you feel your child is ready. Here are some tips:

- The word 'disease' in CD's name can alarm children, so it may be better to talk in terms of a 'poorly tummy' caused by gluten.
- Get children involved in food selection and cooking early. Learning about GF foods can take place during supermarket shopping, meal preparation and outings to restaurants – let them try to choose foods and order their own meals, for instance, and teach them to articulate their requirements to waiting staff.
- Introduce them to new foods regularly – including the unusual ones. Quinoa was the ancient grain of the Incas – build a story, a history lesson, around it to appeal to them.
- Teach them how to decline food. 'No, thank you' may be better than 'I can't eat that.' Teach them that what they put into their bodies is up to them, and there's no obligation to eat something they don't like, even if it is GF or if a relative has 'made it specially'.
- Don't overwhelm children with information at first – issues such as cross-contamination need to be conveyed eventually, but this is something you can manage on their behalf at first.
- Teach them about labelling gradually – the Crossed Grain trade mark is one that they can learn to look out for to help 'break in' to the subject.
- Be positive and upbeat about the situation – your child will pick up on it if you display fretfulness about it. The GFD is absolutely manageable and it's important to convey this to your child.

- Explain CD to other children in the family too. Siblings need to understand the situation and feel involved in the family's care of the coeliac child.
- All kids deserve a treat or reward from time to time, but don't give a coeliac child two treats where you might only give a non-coeliac child one – it's easy to feel you have to offer an extra 'bonus' snack as compensation for having the condition, but ultimately it's not good for the child or the child's tummy.
- If the household is not going GF, it may be helpful to use 'safe' stickers to highlight coeliac-friendly food – you can turn this into an educational game.

Nursery and school

Sending your coeliac child to school can be nerve-racking because suddenly he or she will be under someone else's care and can potentially be exposed to risky foods such as crisps and wheat snacks from other children.

The Coeliac UK website has several parents' school packs, one for each country within the UK, with advice on how to communicate your child's condition to school staff and caterers, and how to work with them to ensure children's needs are provided for. Regional policies differ slightly. For instance, since late 2014, all state-funded schools in England have had to support children with medical conditions, including food sensitivities. The onus is on schools to have policies in place to meet these needs, including health-care plans, and to ensure that these children can participate in all aspects of school life, such as trips away.

Free school lunches should be provided in some circumstances, again dependent on where you live in the UK. If your child takes in a GF packed lunch, you will need to check how closely children are supervised to prevent them swapping foods.

Social events

With regard to after-school activities and children's social clubs, communication is key. Those in charge will be understanding and appreciate the need for vigilance if you convey the seriousness of CD. In situations where children may be given treats, it helps if you supply adults in charge with some GF treats in advance as a standby.

Parties present a bigger problem, as you can't expect other children's parents to serve GF food exclusively. Speak with them well in advance, in person, not on the phone, and offer to supply a GF replacement party parcel for your child, clearly labelled, or to provide a GF cake for the birthday child.

Accept that mistakes will happen and your child may get a little sick. Never punish your child for this. Remember that being 'glutened' may lay your child low for a while, but he or she will get better. Make the best of the bad situation and review the importance of not swapping food or thoughtlessly popping treats into the mouth. Your child is likely to remember the effects of the accident and will instinctively be more careful in future.

Teenagers and CD

Teenagers are rarely diagnosed with CD, so any teenagers with the condition are likely to have had it for some years. At this age, they should be well established on the GFD and understand how to manage their lifestyle. Nevertheless, this is the time during which some teens can get a bit reckless with their diet, possibly as a minor act of rebellion that's sometimes characteristic of this stage of life.

Some teenagers may be curious – 'What does wheat taste like? I wonder if a "real" pizza tastes better than the one I have to eat?' Some succumb to peer pressure – boys especially may be 'dared' to consume a harmful food. Some just get complacent. They may have been well for years. Boys may see themselves as strong and immortal, about to become men, and may feel it isn't macho to 'fuss' about food. They may take risks and may hide it from you, possibly because they don't want you to worry.

It's understandable. Teens want to fit in, not stand out, and they don't want to have to ask to see a label when their mates offer them a sweet from a bag.

The problem with risk-taking is that they may not experience any symptoms. It's a curious fact about the growing teenage coeliac body that it appears adept at not producing overt symptoms of gluten consumption – which is possibly why few are diagnosed at this time. Your son or daughter may feel perfectly well, which could justify and excuse the gluten consumption in his or her mind.

It's worth watching out for any change in health or behaviour and talking to your teen regularly about the GFD in a non-judgemental or castigating way, reminding him or her that damage can be silent, and reiterating the importance of the diet.

But don't get paranoid: many teens manage their GFD and lifestyle with exceptional maturity.

University students

Try not to worry or make too much of a fuss. Equip them with practical things before they set off – toaster bags, some GF supplies, a GF cookbook, their own bread board and biscuit tin. Ensure that they know that they have to communicate their CD to flatmates and fellow students and university caterers. It's pointless to advise most young adults not to drink – but do warn them to stay away from beer (unless GF). A GF food parcel after a few weeks will be warmly received.

10
Staying well

Coeliac disease is a lifelong condition and – at least for the near future – incurable. While the advice in earlier chapters has been mostly focused on getting you or your child better, you need to be aware of how to best stay that way – for life – and overcome any stumbling blocks along the way.

Dietary compliance

It's worth repeating that a strict gluten-free diet is the most important strategy for continuing health and well-being.

Compliance among coeliacs is not always good, and surveys suggest that anywhere between only 45 per cent and 90 per cent stick to the GFD. More at risk of lapses are those who experienced few or only mild symptoms prior to diagnosis.

You should not be reassured by any thoughts of 'safety in numbers' from those percentages – all coeliacs who stray run increased risks of associated short-term and long-term health problems, including abdominal symptoms, poor pregnancy outcomes, nutrient deficiencies and reduced bone mineral density, as well as possibly other autoimmune diseases.

There may be a number of contributory factors to non-compliance:

- Inconvenience – obtaining safe food is more time-consuming, and scanning food labels can be frustrating.
- Cost – specialist gluten-free food is often more expensive.
- Unpalatability – you may miss ordinary bread and pasta, for example, and dislike their replacements.
- Social issues – peer pressure, not wishing to appear different or 'make a fuss'.

- Denial – those with no or few symptoms prior to diagnosis may feel they can 'get away' with consuming occasional gluten as they consider themselves healthy.
- Symptom-free lapses – failure to experience any side effects with gluten intake, whether accidental or deliberate, may reinforce the idea that occasional straying is OK.

Resist any urge to stray. Understand that temptation is likely to come from many sources and inevitably crops up from time to time. Be prepared for situations where it may arise, and remember that all foods have a GF version these days, so you don't need to sacrifice a particular type of food. It's not the bland taste of gluten you're missing or craving – just the familiar one of that sweet or savoury something in which it is found. Support from friends or the online coeliac community can be a great help when you're tempted.

Being 'glutened'

Despite your best intentions, accidents will happen, and you will probably consume some gluten at some point during your GFD, be it through food mistakenly served to you, through cross-contamination or through personal error. Never punish yourself for this. It happens to all.

In some cases, symptoms may be mild, in others very severe. The usual symptom is diarrhoea, often starting the day after, and continuing ill health – perhaps headaches, stomach pain, lethargy – for up to a week or longer. Sometimes the symptoms begin extremely quickly after ingestion. It varies.

Don't make yourself sick if you realize what's happened – this can be dangerous. The deed is done. Rest, eat plain food, perhaps avoiding dairy products for a while, and drink lots of fluids if you have diarrhoea – and ideally a diarrhoea replacement drink too. Some find mint or fennel tea soothing.

There are some digestive enzymes on the market whose manufacturers claim can help with the digestion of gluten and that some coeliacs take when they've inadvertently consumed gluten. Unfortunately, there is insufficient evidence they work and any effects may only be psychological. These enzymes should *never* be used as a means by which to occasionally consume gluten deliberately on the GFD.

Remember that, just like anyone else, coeliacs are prone to upset tummies for other reasons, such as food poisoning, eating rich and spicy foods, eating too much or too fast, consuming too much alcohol with food, or even eating something new that just didn't agree with them. If you do feel 'glutened', it may not always have been gluten.

Continuing symptoms

The gut can take up to two years to heal fully, so don't be surprised if you experience occasional symptoms during the recovery period.

With regard to continuing symptoms, the most common reason is non-compliance with the GFD, either deliberately or unknowingly. In the latter case, try to examine, perhaps over a meeting with your dietitian, whether small amounts of gluten could be sneaking into your diet:

- Are you reading and re-reading labels carefully to make sure foods are GF?
- Have you written a detailed food diary and gone through it with your dietitian to identify possible problems?
- Have you ruled out any cross-contamination possibilities from your kitchen – or other sources?
- Could you be consuming contaminated oats? Or could you be one of the few coeliacs sensitive to even modest portions of GF oats?
- Are you following a diet very high in prescription products made with Codex wheat starch – to which some coeliacs may be sensitive?

The question of a 'safe' level of gluten consumption in coeliacs has not been completely satisfactorily answered, and sensitivity in patients is known to vary.

Studies suggest a long-term daily intake of 10–50 mg of gluten could trigger damage to the gut lining – 500 g of GF bread or pasta at 20 ppm would equate to the lowest level (i.e. 10 mg). Note, though, that this is the most sensitive end of the scale, and that it is unlikely you will consume half a kilogram of GF replacement products a day. Most of those foods will contain much less than 20 ppm of gluten anyway.

Most reactions to Codex wheat starch may not be due to trace gluten protein, but to carbohydrate components instead.

Food sensitivities

Other reactions to foods, perhaps non-permanent ones, may also be a continuing issue in CD, and may be worth considering if accidental gluten intake has been ruled out. The symptoms are usually digestive-based and similar to those found in undiagnosed CD and in irritable bowel syndrome (IBS).

FODMAPs intolerance

FODMAP is an acronym for 'Fermentable Oligosaccharides, Disaccharides, Monosaccharides And Polyols'.

Oligosaccharides, disaccharides, monosaccharides and polyols are four groups of sugars that are generally poorly digested and absorbed in the gut. In many people, this causes no or few problems, but in others, one or more of the four groups may trigger unpleasant symptoms.

The mechanism is quite simple. The sugars pass through the stomach into the small intestine, where they are digested and absorbed to varying degrees. Some sugars are better dealt with than others, and each of us varies in our ability to digest and absorb them – which may change naturally for better or for worse throughout our lifetime, or deteriorate when we are in poor digestive health.

Undigested, unabsorbed FODMAPs continue their journey through the small intestine into the large bowel, or colon. Here, they draw water into the bowel through osmosis and are fermented by beneficial gut bacteria – a perfectly healthy process that produces gas. However, if a lot of water is drawn in, a lot of gas is produced or the bowel is more sensitive, it can all lead, in some individuals, to symptoms of wind, diarrhoea and bloating.

Lactose intolerance

Lactose is a disaccharide sugar – which means it is formed of two (di-) sugar (saccharide) units. In lactose, these two units are glucose and galactose.

Lactose is the sugar found in fresh milk, and it is present to a lesser extent in all other foods made from milk, such as yoghurts and cheeses. Our usual intake is through cows' milk products, but the milk of all mammals, including goats and sheep, also contains lactose.

The digestive enzyme that breaks down lactose is called lactase, and this is produced in the tips of the villi that line the small intestine. Damage to your gut lining caused by previously undiagnosed CD may mean that your body's ability to produce lactase is hampered, and so the lactose you consume remains undigested and unabsorbed – leading to abdominal pain, gas and frothy diarrhoea, typically half an hour or more after the consumption of some dairy products.

A hydrogen breath test (HBT) for lactose intolerance is available; it measures hydrogen levels in your breath following consumption of milk – an indicator of intolerance. If confirmed, you will generally need to avoid milk, ice cream, custards, creams, soft cheeses and perhaps other dairy products, depending on your sensitivity, which you'll usually be able to gauge by trial and error.

Yoghurts, butter and hard or mature cheeses tend to be much lower in lactose and may be tolerated well. It is better to eat these foods with other foods, rather than on an empty stomach, as they will be better tolerated.

Low-lactose milks and other dairy products are available, and there are plenty of vegan milks – such as nut, soya or rice milks – and related products too. Alternative sources of calcium (see pp. 70–71) must be included if lactose intolerance is severe enough to warrant a dairy-free or reduced-diary diet.

As one of the 14 key allergens, milk or milk-based ingredients must be emphasized on food labelling. Some GF products are additionally dairy free, but this may not be flagged as prominently as their GF status.

Lactose intolerance caused by CD is usually temporary but, in some cases, may last for a year or more even on the GFD, until the gut heals sufficiently and the ability to produce lactase is restored. You can try to increase or reintroduce lactose-containing foods gradually over time, perhaps under the guidance of your dietitian, and this in itself may help to 'retrain' your system to accept lactose again.

Fructose intolerance or malabsorption

Fructose, like glucose, is a monosaccharide – which means it is formed of a single (mono-) sugar unit. Unlike glucose, though, it is poorly absorbed by the body, and those with digestive problems such as CD may have greater difficulty than others absorbing it. The resulting symptoms are similar to those in lactose intolerance, and again an HBT may help identify the intolerance.

Fructose is also found in table sugar – the disaccharide sucrose – in which it is bound with glucose. In this form it does not trigger symptoms. It is 'free' fructose – in excess of glucose – that seems problematic. There are several rich sources of such fructose in the diet, among which are:

- many fruits (e.g. apples, mango, watermelons, pears, black currants, cherries), their juices and concentrates, and some dried fruit;
- corn, high-fructose or sugar syrups; some jams; honey and treacle;
- fortified wines;
- some sports or energy drinks.

Malabsorption of polyols

Sometimes called the sugar alcohols – although they are not alcoholic in the usual sense – the polyols include sorbitol, maltitol, mannitol, xylitol and isomalt. They are very poorly absorbed. They are used as sweeteners and tend to be found in slimming drinks and diet foods, chewing gum, low-sugar soft drinks and diabetic foods.

But they are naturally found in mushrooms, and some fruits and their juices too: for instance, sorbitol is in apples, pears, avocado and stone fruit (e.g. plums, apricot, cherries) and xylitol in berries.

Malabsorption of oligosaccharides

'Oligos' means few or several, and the oligosaccharides are formed of three or more sugar units. They are particularly poorly digested and absorbed by all of us. There are two types of relevance to our diets:

- Fructo-oligosaccharides (FOS), and a similar class of carbo-hydrates called inulins, consist largely of a number of joined fructose sugar units – key dietary sources are wheat starch, the allium vegetables (onion, garlic, leek), artichokes (globe, and especially Jerusalem), asparagus, beetroot and chicory.
- Galacto-oligosaccharides (GOS) consist largely of several joined galactose sugar units – the key sources are beans and pulses, hummus and some nuts (cashews, pistachios).

The pity with regard to these poorly absorbed sugars is that they happen to be good for us. They act as prebiotics, feeding beneficial bacteria in the gut, help with calcium absorption, and are even thought to protect against bowel cancer – among other benefits. (FOS and GOS are sometimes referred to as fructans and galactans, respectively.)

Some low-FODMAP GF foods

This is a small selection. FODMAP content of foods is still being researched, and may vary according to its species, the climate or soil in which it is grown, its culinary preparation, its ripeness and other factors. Data for some foods are not publicly available, and as FODMAP research is a relatively new 'science', lists are subject to change.

- Vegetables: some green vegetables (kale, spinach, green beans), salad vegetables (lettuce, tomatoes, cucumber, radish), root vegetables (carrot, potato, turnip, parsnip), Mediterranean vegetables (courgette, peppers, aubergine, fennel)
- Fruit: citrus fruit, melons other than watermelon, grapes, strawberries
- Meats and seafood
- Grains: rice, GF oats, millet, buckwheat, amaranth, quinoa and most products made from them or their flours, such as pastas
- Most condiments and sauces, most dressings
- Tofu and tempeh
- Mature cheeses, butter, eggs
- Dark chocolate.

Diagnosing a FODMAP problem

Diagnosing an intolerance to the simpler FODMAPs is by means of an HBT, but many individuals are able to cope well enough with normal quantities of lactose and fructose. Others 'instinctively' limit their milk intake, for example, almost subconsciously, to their personal threshold.

The more complex FODMAPs can be trickier to pin down – and are also perhaps more likely to be the culprits of continuing symptoms, especially the oligosaccharides.

Your dietitian may think a low-FODMAP elimination diet is worth attempting. Never go it alone as it is restrictive, complicated and difficult to follow, and nutritional deficiencies (in particular, of calcium) are possible. It also requires a dietitian trained in FODMAPs to interpret it properly.

It is a diagnostic test diet from which suspect foods are first removed for up to eight weeks. If symptoms persist beyond that period, the problem may be psychological, not FODMAPs-related, or not food-related at all.

If symptoms clear, the reintroduction phase can begin, where groups are individually and gradually brought back into the diet in order to monitor any reactions. The reintroduction of a food followed by the return of symptoms may point to an intolerance to a particular food or FODMAP. It is unlikely that the food will need to be completely avoided: working with your dietitian can often help you discover a modest tolerance threshold.

Some patients reintroduce all foods without problems – a change of diet can sometimes be all that's needed to clear up symptoms.

Going it alone

Some cautious and 'light' dietary experimentation is unlikely to require dietetic support or compromise health. Wheat (in large amounts), onions and garlic are commonly found to be problematic foods, so if you rely heavily on prescription goods with Codex wheat starch in them and eat a lot of allium vegetables, consider cutting back for a while to see whether you experience benefit. The same goes for any other particular food you may recognize from the high-FODMAP lists that you consume a lot of – for instance, sugar-free gum or very large quantities of fruit or juices.

Do not make wholesale dietary changes or experiment drastically on your own.

Food allergy

The most common type of food allergy – called IgE-mediated food allergy – is well known: it causes symptoms such as wheezing, itchy mouth and lips, rashes, swelling to the face, nausea and other symptoms that come on quickly after eating the offending food. Peanuts, nuts, eggs and fish are common triggers. This form may well co-exist with CD, but cannot be mistaken for continuing bowel-related symptoms.

However, there is another type of allergy – non-IgE-mediated food allergy – in which the symptoms are typically restricted to the digestive system and skin (reflux, heartburn, diarrhoea, eczema, itchiness) and are delayed, not immediate. It is much rarer, and an unlikely cause, but one that may be worth exploring with your dietitian via an elimination diet, as blood tests aren't available. It may be caused by meats, seafood, soya, milk, nuts or other foods.

Other food sensitivities

There are many unusual reactions to foods, food ingredients and natural food chemicals beyond the scope of this book.

Reactions to glycoalkaloids (in nightshade vegetables such as tomatoes, potatoes), oxalates (in rhubarb, beetroot, chard), lectins (in beans and pulses) and other chemicals may trigger gastrointestinal symptoms in susceptible individuals – as might the preservatives (especially sulphites), sweeteners or flavour enhancers routinely used in processed food these days. There may be a case for exploring rarer possibilities with your dietitian.

Some with 'sensitive guts' may react to fatty foods, very high fibre foods, coffee (especially on an empty stomach), spices and (GF) beer. Experimenting with cutting back on these if you consume them in large amounts may be worthwhile.

You may be tempted by private 'allergy' or 'intolerance' tests for idiosyncratic food sensitivities, even when marketed by high street outlets, but avoid all those described on pp. 24–25 as they are unvalidated.

Continuing problems: other possibilities

There are a few other possible causes of persistent symptoms.

Irritable bowel syndrome

A 'collection of otherwise unexplained symptoms relating to a disturbance of the colon or large intestine' is how the IBS Network define irritable bowel syndrome (IBS). It is common in the general population, and can co-exist with CD. Often it is linked to stress. It is not a disease.

As well as a wide catalogue of bowel symptoms, those with IBS may experience headaches, muscular pains, tiredness, indigestion and other symptoms.

Around 10 per cent of coeliacs who don't respond to the GFD may have underlying IBS too, and it is possible that the symptoms they were experiencing that led to their coeliac diagnosis may actually have been caused by undiagnosed IBS, while their CD was asymptomatic all along.

IBS can be diagnosed only by your doctor. He or she may wish to exclude other possibilities first, and some tests may be required.

Your doctor or dietitian may advise adjustments to your fibre intake, perhaps reducing insoluble fibre (e.g. brown rice, fruit and vegetable skins, nuts) and increasing soluble fibre (e.g. fruit and vegetables). Other dietary modifications may help – including a reduced-FODMAP diet, which research has shown to be promising in managing IBS symptoms in around 75 per cent of patients when supported by a dietitian. But what works for one person will not work for another, so advice must be individualized.

Some general tips are to eat at regular intervals and not to skip meals, and to reduce intake of caffeinated, fizzy or alcoholic drinks. Eating five small meals may be better than eating three larger ones. Take your time; eat slowly.

Anti-spasmodic medication may be recommended, and relaxation therapy and hypnotherapy have been shown to help.

There is more in my book, *IBS: Dietary Advice to Calm Your Gut*, co-authored with dietitian Julie Thompson.

Small intestinal bacterial overgrowth

Small intestinal bacterial overgrowth (SIBO), or small bowel bacterial overgrowth (SBBO), is a condition in which there is an excess of bacteria in the small intestine, leading to symptoms of diarrhoea, wind, pain and bloating. According to the British Society of Gastroenterology, it is underdiagnosed in the population and may well occur in some coeliac patients who have continuing problems despite a GFD. It appears to be more common in those with diabetes or Crohn's disease and may account for some IBS cases.

It can be diagnosed via an HBT, and antibiotics are the usual course of treatment. Taking probiotics (see p. 76) may offer some benefits too, as may reducing your sugar intake, but check with your doctor or dietitian first.

Pancreatic insufficiency

This is the inability to properly digest food as a result of poor production of digestive enzymes by the pancreas. Symptoms include fatty diarrhoea or floating stools, wind, bloating and weight loss. It may result in poor absorption of food, and subsequent symptoms of tiredness and malnutrition caused by anaemia. It has been proposed as a not uncommon problem in CD patients with persistent symptoms. It is more likely if you also have type 1 diabetes. It can be diagnosed via a stool test, possibly along with other tests, and the treatment is enzyme supplementation.

Bile acid malabsorption (BAM)

Bile acids are produced by the liver to aid digestion, and in a healthy small intestine should be reabsorbed back into the system. But any damage to the portion of small intestine responsible for this – perhaps caused by surgery, CD, Crohn's disease or SIBO – may mean it doesn't occur. The bile salts reach the large intestine, draw in water and trigger urgent, pale or greasy diarrhoea. BAM is diagnosed via a scan (called SeHCAT), and medication will be prescribed.

Poor diet

Is your GFD healthy? It's an important question, one that you should answer honestly. It can be tempting to comfort eat after a coeliac diagnosis, but your diet needs to be balanced in order to encourage recovery at a time when your gut lining is trying to heal. You need nourishing and nutrient-dense foods. Home-cooked meals are best. Avoid excess sweet foods, which could lead to problems with FODMAP absorption. See Chapter 5 for healthy eating advice.

Misdiagnosis

It is possible for people to be misdiagnosed with CD when they don't have it, but this is rare these days owing to advances in diagnostic procedures and awareness. However, if you were diagnosed prior to the turn of the millennium, it may be worth discussing this outside possibility with your medical team if all else has been ruled out.

Other autoimmune conditions

These are discussed in Chapter 6 and may need to be investigated.

Aftercare

It's vital that you accept follow-up care, as research shows it helps you to stick to a GFD. It also allows you to discuss and hopefully resolve any problems.

The level of aftercare offered to you by the health service will vary according to region, and there are few guidelines and some mixed views on who you should see – and how often. Do not be afraid to ask.

A lack of local resources may mean you don't receive the level of aftercare you would like. See your doctor or speak to Coeliac

UK if this is a problem in your area or if you are left largely to manage on your own. At the very least, you should receive an annual review.

Your dietitian

Ideally, you should have regular follow-up appointments with your dietitian or paediatric dietitian in the first year following diagnosis if you need them. This is helpful for reviewing your progress and your understanding of the GFD, for untangling any sticking points and for addressing any continuing nutritional problems. Your dietitian can also help with any struggles to maintain your GFD and continuing symptoms – perhaps by checking your understanding of food labelling or by ordering further tests.

Children must be closely monitored and examined to ensure that their development and growth progress normally. A dietary assessment by a paediatric dietitian can help to identify nutritional deficiencies and any need for supplements.

Your GP

Use your GP as a continuing source of health advice and support – he or she can help with your prescriptions, with arranging or performing further tests, and with vaccinations such as for pneumococcal disease and influenza, and may also conduct your annual follow-up and assessment.

Follow-up tests

There are several follow-up tests that you may need.

Blood tests

A full blood count and a check of nutrient levels – iron, calcium, B vitamins, etc. – should ideally be performed every year, and more regularly under particular circumstances.

Coeliac antibody tests may be repeated as regularly, to check that the levels of antibodies to tissue transglutaminase have reduced (see p. 18). In children, it is recommended that these tests be performed after six months of a GFD. In practice, children dislike giving blood, and if the consultant believes recovery is strong after several years, blood tests may not always be performed unless there is a specific concern.

Liver or thyroid function tests may be appropriate.

DEXA bone scan

Those with abnormal bone density should be reassessed every three years. Children are unlikely to require a DEXA scan.

Endoscopy and biopsy

These may be advised in certain circumstances, for instance to check that the gut lining is healing, or to confirm an uncertain diagnosis (often in children), or to examine whether oat reintroduction has triggered villous atrophy.

Serious complications

These are very rare in CD but do occur.

Refractory CD is CD in which the gut does not heal on a strict GFD. One form can be treated with corticosteroids and the prognosis is good, but the second form is more serious and lymphoma (cancer) of the intestine usually follows, which has a poor prognosis.

There is a very slightly increased chance of other malignancies of the gastrointestinal tract among newly diagnosed patients with CD, but once someone has been established on the GFD for several years, the risk is equivalent to that of a non-coeliac.

11
The outlook

Alternatives to the gluten-free diet are needed, largely because the diet is expensive and difficult and because compliance with it is sometimes poor. Further, coeliac disease is on the rise worldwide and there is concern that this will increasingly burden health-care providers, adding to the demands placed upon them by low diagnosis rates.

Future treatments

There are four possibilities:

1 Treatments that work in addition to a GFD
2 Treatments that minimize possible health effects of hidden, trace or accidentally consumed gluten in the GFD
3 Treatments that allow moderate gluten consumption
4 Treatments that replace the GFD and allow a regular diet.

There are various treatments that are being proposed, developed and trialled, and some are considered below. It may not be until the mid-2020s that one or more will become widely available commercially. Some may fail at trial stage if, for instance, unacceptable side effects are encountered, but even a single viable one could transform lives – even if only by offering greater peace of mind and reduced risk of the possible effects of cross-contamination when dining out.

Vaccine therapy

Of the many thousands of protein parts (called peptides) found in gluten, the bulk of the immune response activated in CD is caused by just three, and it is these three that are most toxic to coeliacs. From this starting point, scientists at the Walter and

Eliza Hall Institute in Melbourne, Australia, led by Dr Robert Anderson, developed a potential vaccine, Nexvax2, synthesized to work by 'introducing' these fragments of gluten to the immune system of coeliacs in a particular way, 're-educating' them to tolerate the protein and not to react inappropriately. Sadly, in 2019, a phase 2 trial failed to demonstrate any protection from gluten exposure in coeliac patients given the vaccine, and the trial was halted prematurely. It was a major setback, and the future of Nexvax2 and other therapeutic vaccines is now uncertain.

However, vaccine therapy may have a role in CD prevention. Children genetically predisposed to CD appear more likely to develop it after a rotavirus infection – a vaccine against this may offer some protection in a subset of infants.

Enzyme therapy

A gluten enzyme called Latiglutenase has been designed to help break down gluten into non-toxic fragments in the stomach. It is designed only to offer protection against the accidental ingestion of very small amounts of gluten – such as through cross-contamination – which are difficult to avoid when following a GFD.

Another enzyme, called KumaMax, has been shown capable of breaking down 95 per cent of a toxic gluten peptide.

Trials for both are ongoing.

Helminthic therapy

Not for the squeamish, this involves inoculating CD patients with a harmless hookworm to interfere with immune responses and alter responsivity to gluten. This is based on the idea that our sterile Western modes of living and antibiotic-rich medicine cabinets, which have eradicated intestinal parasitic worms from our bodies, have detrimentally affected our immune responses, increasing the tendency towards autoimmune conditions. Kept 'distracted' by these parasites, the immune system ignores the 'threat' of gluten. It has shown great promise in a few trials, with some individuals being able to reintroduce modest portions of gluten-containing foods for a short period.

Drug therapy

INN-202 (larazotide acetate) is a drug that blocks the action of zonulin, a protein that 'unlocks' the intestinal barrier and increases the gut's permeability, or leakiness, to gluten fragments. Those with autoimmune disease produce higher levels of zonulin. When taken before a meal, INN-202 may help 'shore up' the gut lining to protect it against an inflammatory response to gluten.

BL-7010 is a drug which works by binding to gluten, thereby reducing its toxicity, and carrying it out of the system.

ZED1227 is a drug which blocks tissue transglutaminase (tTG), an enzyme in the body which reacts with gluten and enhances its inflammatory capabilities. Suppressing this could prevent the immune response.

These are currently being trialled, as are several others, including drugs for refractory CD.

Stem cell therapy

An exciting potential therapy is one that would involve stem cell transplantations, perhaps from a sibling, to cure CD. There are several experimental cases on record with reasonably good reported outcomes, but more research and clinical trials are needed.

Future 'free from' foods

Some experts and coeliac patients feel that research and investment would be better geared towards the development of improved and more innovative 'free from' products – as opposed to medical treatments.

Genetic modification of wheat is potentially revolutionary, albeit controversial. Some researchers have suggested it may be possible to 'breed out' the toxic elements of gluten, and others are working on ways to 'disable' them or otherwise 'hide' them from the immune system, effectively producing a wheat safe for those with CD.

There is evidence to suggest different oat cultivars have variable levels of toxicity, with the potential for one or two to be safe for all.

The use of *Lactobacillus* bacteria in sourdough bread has been arousing interest for some time: it appears that these bacteria can break down toxic gluten peptides to some extent, rendering the bread 'safer', but further studies and development are needed.

Other protein enzymes – called proteases – may also have potential in the development of new 'free from' foods, serving to 'pre-digest' gluten in order to formulate more palatable products.

Food technology is moving in unusual directions: combining proteins from the blood of cows with saccharides (sugars), for example, has been found to improve the texture of GF bread.

Foods are needed that tackle the metabolic disorders and health problems CD patients often have to deal with: higher-calcium breads for patients who avoid milk due to lactose intolerance, for instance, and low GI (glycaemic index) foods to address obesity (see p. 75). Low-FODMAP GF foods could be next 'big thing' in the 'free from' aisle.

Future testing and diagnoses

More specific and sensitive blood tests – and, potentially, less invasive urine tests – may eventually render the biopsy redundant, although some specialists feel it should be retained. An accurate blood test that requires the patient to spend considerably less time on a gluten-containing diet is being looked at.

A test for avenin (oat protein) sensitivity in CD would be a breakthrough, and is being explored.

The more we learn about the genes associated with autoimmune conditions, the more we may be able to predict those destined to develop CD, including children, and perhaps eventually take preventative action.

The question of universal screening remains unsettled. With half a million undiagnosed cases in the UK, some have argued a coeliac test should become as routine as a cholesterol test. On the other hand, there is the moral concern that it would 'impose' disease on people who may consider themselves healthy and not wish to know otherwise. The burden on health care must also be considered.

Onwards ...

Never before have gluten-related disorders been the subject of so much attention or been so visible in the public domain. As scientists and researchers continue to do extraordinary work in the field, it is impossible to predict what the future may be. What we must hope for is that the conspicuous profile of CD and gluten-related disorders proves beneficial to generations both present and future.

Useful addresses

Coeliac charities

Coeliac UK
  Third Floor, Apollo Centre
  Desborough Road
  High Wycombe
  Bucks HP11 2QW
  Tel: 01494 437278
  Helpline: 0333 332 2033
  Website: www.coeliac.org.uk

  Scotland office:
  Regus
  83 Princes Street
  Edinburgh EH2 2ER
  Tel: 0131 357 4614

  Wales office:
  Heritage House
  Fitzalan Place
  Cardiff CF24 0BL
  Tel: 029 2049 9732

Coeliac Society of Ireland
  Carmichael House
  4 North Brunswick Street
  Dublin 7
  Tel.: +353 1 872 1471
  Website: www.coeliac.ie

Other UK health organizations

British Sjögren's Syndrome Association
  Tel.: 0121 478 1133
  Website: www.bssa.uk.net

British Society of Gastroenterology
  Tel.: 020 7935 3150
  Website: www.bsg.org.uk

British Thyroid Foundation
  Tel.: 01423 810093
  Website: www.btf-thyroid.org

Core (gut/liver/pancreas health charity)
  Tel.: 020 7486 0341
  Website: www.corecharity.org.uk

Crohn's and Colitis UK
  Tel.: 0300 222 5700 (helpline)
  Website: www.crohnsandcolitis.org.uk

Diabetes UK
  Tel.: 0345 123 2399 (helpline)
  Website: www.diabetes.org.uk

The IBS Network
  Tel.: 0114 272 3253
  Website: www.theibsnetwork.org

Multiple Sclerosis Society
  Tel.: 0808 800 8000
  Website: www.mssociety.org.uk

Royal Osteoporosis Society
  Tel.: 0808 800 0035 (helpline)
  Website: www.nos.org.uk

Informational sites and blogs

Many of these include links to dozens of other useful sites.

  Alex Gazzola's blog: www.allergy-insight.com

  The Coeliactivist: www.coeliactivist.com

  Coeliac Sanctuary: www.coeliacsanctuary.co.uk

  Foods Matter: www.foodsmatter.com

  Glutarama: www.glutarama.com

Gluten Free Alchemist: www.glutenfreealchemist.com

Gluten Free Ireland: www.glutenfreeireland.com

Gluten Free Mrs D: www.glutenfreemrsd.com

NHS Choices (CD pages): www.nhs.uk/conditions/coeliac-disease

NICE (CD guidelines): www.nice.org.uk/ng20

NICE (CD quality standard): www.nice.org.uk/guidance/QS134

'Free from' food manufacturers

Below is a small selection. Links to many others can be found at www.allergy-insight.com/free-from-food. All supermarkets, though not listed here, also have own-brand 'free from' ranges, and can send lists of GF own-brand products.

* denotes prescription supplier.

Amy's Kitchen (www.amyskitchen.co.uk)
Soups and ready-meals

BFree Foods (www.bfreefoods.com)
Breads, wraps, rolls

Delicious Alchemy (www.deliciousalchemy.com)
Bakery mixes, cereals

Doves Farm (www.dovesfarm.co.uk)
Pasta, flours, baked goods, cereals

Drossa UK Ltd* (www.drossa.co.uk)
Pasta, gnocchi, bakery mixes

Free From Italy (www.freefromitaly.co.uk)
Pastas, breads, gnocchi, sauces

Genius Gluten Free* (www.geniusglutenfree.com)
Baked goods, pastas

Glebe Farm (www.glebe-flour.co.uk)
Flours, cakes, mixes, cereals, oat milk

Glutafin* (www.glutafin.co.uk)
Bakery, flour mixes, pastas, crackers, cereal, pizza bases

Gluten Free Foods Ltd* (www.glutenfree-foods.co.uk)
Barkat breads, pasta, flour mixes, snacks, biscuits, cakes, cereals

Gosh! Food (www.goshfood.com)
Vegan sausages, burgers and bites

Green's (www.glutenfreebeers.co.uk)
GF beers

Innovative Solutions UK Ltd* (www.pureglutenfree.co.uk)
Pure flours, baking ingredients

Juvela* (www.juvela.co.uk)
Breads, pasta, pizza bases, flour mixes, crackers, biscuits, cereals

Kelkin (www.kelkin.ie)
Bakery, cereal, pasta, biscuits: in the UK and the Republic of Ireland

Mrs Crimble's (www.mrscrimbles.com)
Breads, mixes, crackers, cakes, sweet treats

Nairn's* (www.nairns-oatcakes.com)
GF oat crackers, flatbreads, snacks, biscuits and cereals

Orgran* (www.orgranglutenfree.co.uk)
Pasta, crispbreads, cereals, biscuits, snacks, bread/flour mixes

Rizopia* (www.rizopia.co.uk)
Pastas

Schär (www.schaer.com/en-uk)
Bakery, snacks, pizza, ready meals

Warburtons Gluten Free* (www.warburtonsglutenfree.com)
Breads and wraps

Apps

Foodmaestro Food Finder – free to download, 'for people with allergies and / or lifestyle restrictions'. See www.foodmaestro.me

Gluten Free Food Checker App – available free to all Coeliac UK members, and downloadable from the Apple App or Google Play stores. App includes a barcode scanner, lists of ingredients and nutritional info, and facility to add other declarable or 'top 14' allergens. Search for it on www.coeliac.org.uk

Social media

Some of the key organizations mentioned in this resources section have active chat forums, and most have social media accounts, including Facebook (which hosts dozens of coeliac-related public and private groups) and Twitter, which is an excellent source of news. In the latter, hashtags regularly used in coeliac-related conversations include, among others, #coeliac, #celiac and #glutenfree.

Alex Gazzola: www.twitter.com/HealthJourno and www.facebook.com/HealthJourno

Coeliac UK: www.twitter.com/coeliac_uk and www.facebook.com/coeliacuk

The Coeliac, DH and Gluten Free Message Board: http://members2.boardhost.com/glutenfree

Annual events / shows

Many local GF fairs take place throughout the year; your local coeliac group should have information. The Coeliac UK website will also have details of conferences and scientific meetings, sometimes open to members of the public. The Coeliac Society of Ireland hold The Gluten Free Living Show in Dublin in autumn.

The Allergy & Free From Show (UK)
www.allergyshow.co.uk
Three shows (London, Liverpool, Glasgow) taking place each year, open to the public, featuring hundreds of exhibitors, many of them GF.

The Free From Food Awards (UK)
www.freefromfoodawards.co.uk
Annual awards for free from foods, including GF. Invitation-only ceremony held in Spring.

Free From Festival (UK)
www.freefromfestival.co.uk

Shows in several cities in the UK, showcasing artisanal and smaller GF and dairy-free food and drink producers.

North American coeliac organizations

Beyond Celiac: www.beyondceliac.org

Canadian Celiac Association: www.celiac.ca

Celiac Disease Foundation: www.celiac.org

Gluten Intolerance Group: www.gluten.org

National Celiac Association: www.nationalceliac.org

US coeliac disease centres

The University of Chicago Celiac Disease Center: www.cureceliacdisease.org

Columbia University Celiac Disease Center: www.celiacdiseasecenter.columbia.edu

Other international coeliac groups

Many non-anglophone nations' sites offer English-language advice for visitors.

Europe

Österreichische Arbeitsgemeinschaft Zöliakie (Austria): www.zoeliakie.or.at

Vlaamse Coeliakie Vereniging (Belgium – Flemish-speaking): www.coeliakie.be

Société Belge de la Coeliaquie (Belgium – French-speaking): www.vivresansgluten.be

Hrvatsko Društvo za Celijakiju (Croatia): www.celijakija.hr

Společnost pro bezlepkovou dietu (Czech Republic): http://celiak.cz/en

Dansk Cøliaki Forening (Denmark): www.coeliaki.dk

Keliakialiitto (Finland): www.keliakialiitto.fi

Association Française des Intolérants au Gluten (France): www.afdiag.fr

Deutsche Zöliakiegesellschaft (Germany): www.dzg-online.de

Greek Coeliac Society: www.koiliokaki.com

Lisztérzékenyek Érdekképviseletének Országos Egyesülete (Hungary): www.coeliac.hu/tiki-index.php

Associazione Italiana Celiachia (Italy): www.celiachia.it

Nederlandse Coeliakie Vereniging (Netherlands): www.glutenvrij.nl

Norsk Cøliakiforening (Norway): www.ncf.no

Polskie Stowarzyszenie Osøb z Celiakia i Na Diecie Bezglutenowej (Poland): www.celiakia.org.pl

Associação Portuguesa de Celíacos (Portugal): www.celiacos.org.pt

Celiakia (Slovakia): www.celiakia.sk

Slovensko Društvo za Celiakijo (Slovenia): www.drustvo-celiakija.si

Federación de Asociaciones de Celíacos de España (Spain): www.celiacos.org

Svenska Celiakiförbundet (Sweden): www.celiaki.se

IC Zöliakie der Deutschen Schweiz (Switzerland): www.zoeliakie.ch

Asia and Oceania

The Coeliac Society of Australia: www.coeliac.org.au

The Israeli Celiac Association: www.celiac.org.il

Coeliac New Zealand: www.coeliac.org.nz

Çölyakla Yaşam Derneği (Turkey): www.colyak.org.tr

Further reading

Gluten-free directories

In the UK
Food and Drink Guide, produced annually by Coeliac UK

In Ireland
Food List, produced annually by the Coeliac Society of Ireland

Books

Fasano, Alessio and Flaherty, Susie, *Gluten Freedom*, Nashville, Tennessee: Turner Publishing, 2014

Gazzola, Alex and Thompson Julie, *IBS: Dietary Advice to Calm Your Gut*, Sheldon Press, 2017

Print magazines

Allergic Living (Canada): www.allergicliving.com

Australian Gluten-Free Life (Aus): www.agfl.com.au

Delight Gluten Free (USA): www.delightglutenfree.com

Gluten Free and More (USA): www.glutenfreeandmore.com

Gluten-Free Living (USA): www.glutenfreeliving.com

Live Well Gluten Free (UK): www.coeliac.org.uk

Simply Gluten Free (USA): www.simplygluten-free.com

Recipe books

Devlin, Naomi, *River Cottage Gluten Free*, Bloomsbury Publishing, 2016

Devonshire, Jane, *Hassle Free, Gluten Free*, Absolute Press, 2018

Kendrick, Pippa, *Free From Food for Family and Friends*, London: HarperCollins, 2014

Vickery, Phil, *Essential Gluten Free*, Kyle Books, 2016

Index

Overcoming Common Problems Series

Selected titles

A full list of titles is available from Sheldon Press on our
website at www.sheldonpress.co.uk

Lists of titles in the Mindful Way and Sheldon Short Guides series are also available from Sheldon Press.

Alex Gazzola is a health journalist who has written for over a hundred

The item should be returned or renewed by the last date stamped below.

Dylid dychwelyd neu adnewyddu'r eitem erbyn y dyddiad olaf sydd wedi'i stampio isod. *Cent*

To renew visit / Adnewyddwch ar
www.newport.gov.uk/libraries